Praise for

A FIELD GUIDE TO
BUYING ORGANIC

"All organic food is not created equal. *A Field Guide to Buying Organic* answers questions about when you should buy organic and when you should skip it."
—*Baltimore Sun*

"If you're still trying to decide whether you should go organic, pick up *A Field Guide to Buying Organic*. Whatever your questions about organics—how they compare in price to their conventional counterparts, their availability, etc.—chances are the answers are in this book."—*Health*

"Luddene Perry and Dan Schultz's new book will tell you how to navigate the aisles by deciphering the numerous—and often vague—declarations that adorn grocery products. By delving into the science and machinations behind the organic-food movement, they'll help you figure out what you want too."
—*Time Out New York* (Critic's Pick)

A FIELD GUIDE TO

BUYING
ORGANIC

A FIELD GUIDE TO
BUYING
ORGANIC

■

Luddene Perry &

Dan Schultz

Bantam Books

A FIELD GUIDE TO BUYING ORGANIC
A Bantam Book

PUBLISHING HISTORY
Bantam trade paperback edition published September 2005
Bantam mass market edition / February 2007

Published by
Bantam Dell
A Division of Random House, Inc.
New York, New York

Book design by Robert Bull

Library of Congress Catalog Card Number: 2005048267

ISBN 978-0-553-59029-6

Printed in the United States of America
Published simultaneously in Canada

www.bantamdell.com

OPM 10 9 8 7 6 5

Contents

Acknowledgments

It is not possible to truly acknowledge everyone who contributed in their own ways to the writing of this book, but a number of people deserve special recognition.

On a personal note, we would both like to thank Therese Jacobs-Stewart and Jim Jacobs: without them, this book would never have happened.

Luddene would like to thank Lisa Harmony, for her willingness to listen; Michael Saeger, for his honest critique; and John and Nancy Bierbaum, for their generosity and support.

Dan remains indebted to Shari Hess, John and Carolyn Schultz, Andrew and Kari Schultz, Steve Schwandt, Gary Ukura, Berenice Hillion, Erik Haugo, and Carolyn Hess.

Special thanks to our agent, Laura Friedman Williams, for her insights, her patience, and her always timely, encouraging words; and to everyone at Bantam, especially our editor, Philip Rappaport, who continually challenged us to imagine a better book.

Thanks also to Angie Bertrand, for her graphic-saving grace.

And to numerous others who, unbeknownst to them, offered kind and helpful thoughts along the way.

A FIELD GUIDE TO
BUYING ORGANIC

Introduction

Is organic food worth it?

It seems like a simple question, usually delivered in a way that reveals the questioner's preconceived notion of the answer. Although there's always an emphasis on *worth,* the *it* is the litmus test. The believer in organic food uses *it* as an eye-narrowing challenge. The skeptic tosses *it* away. And the simply curious hold *it* up, for examination—like an apple—in the light.

Our answer is always the same: It depends.

Yes, but is organic food worth it?

In the spirit of the curious, we set out to answer the question. We too had our preconceived notions, and we filled our offices with sources from both sides of the aisle. Most of the literature we could find took a strong position— either enthusiastically pro-organic or sarcastically against it. We have written the book we couldn't find.

Our idea, at first, was simple: I would offer my thirty-five years of organic experience, and Dan would serve as both a foil and a stand-in for consumers increasingly removed from the soil and the realities of food production.

He was well suited to the task. In addition to having a lifelong love of fresh produce from his grandparents' farm, Dan supplemented his teaching salary with a summer job as a pest-control operator, fumigating flour mills and grain elevators. Despite his experiences on the farm and in the conventional food industry, he—like many people—knew very little about what happens to food before it becomes a mosaic of colorful packages on a supermarket shelf.

For me, the task was a chance to walk down my own organic memory lane back to J. I. Rodale and *Organic Farming and Gardening* magazine. When the first issue came out in May 1942, industrial agriculture had already established itself as the future of food production, but Rodale saw a different future, extolling the virtues and value of compost—"black gold," he called it. I bought my first copy in 1968, and Rodale's romantic descriptions of the organic gardening life echoed my own fond memories of my grandmother's farm, of me perched on a bale of hay in the predawn light watching her milk our Jersey cow.

In 1968 growing food without chemicals was fast becoming a political act, but I just wanted to have a great garden and be as self-sufficient as possible. At the time, I didn't know much about fertilizers or pesticides, but I understood Rodale's idea: restore the soil with compost, and you wouldn't need them. That was the promise, and I was hooked before I finished the first issue.

In the decades that followed, organic foods moved from the backyard to the commune to the co-op, and I was involved every step of the way—from gardening to inspecting to certifying. By 1982 I had decided to devote my life to organic production practices and pursued a master's degree in horticultural food production, then started a Ph.D. in agriculture waste management. I didn't finish it, but I know more about manure than I dare discuss at a cocktail party.

Today organic food is a multibillion-dollar industry largely controlled by corporations and regulated by the U.S. Department of Agriculture (USDA). With a 15 to 20 percent growth rate, organic food is the agricultural equivalent of striking oil. Black gold indeed. And when you consider that organics currently makes up just 2 percent of the entire food industry, it isn't too much of a stretch to imagine the enthusiastic salivation taking place in corporate boardrooms.

Of course, not everyone is happy about this development. Rodale's compost has fertilized the growth of a number of organic ideologies, from mom-and-pop principles to the politics of big business.

The promise of organics—or some version of it anyway—has become a reality. Gone are the bins full of oats and the wormy apples common in the pre-supermarket era. Today shoppers push carts past pleasant displays of organic food, guided by friendly store personnel who dutifully explain the virtues of higher-priced organic food.

But is organic food worth it?

It depends.

To buy or not to buy has become the question in household debates that touch on issues central to our lives: our health, the environment, social justice, and the family budget. Overall, these discussions are fortified with limited and bewildering information. We may believe there are good reasons to buy organic food, but what exactly are those reasons?

By providing the necessary background to make informed decisions, *A Field Guide to Buying Organic* encourages you to define your own organic ethic. We've done some digging in order to frame the issues and help you make thoughtful decisions about your food budget, but our goal is to inform, not to preach. For some, this information will stimulate interest in buying organic. Others may become more skeptical. Whatever your reaction, you will be free to develop your own ideas about the value of organic foods, because we have found that the question of worth leaves out the most important element: *It depends on you.*

In short, this book does not accept at face value all the claims made about organic products; nor does it excuse concerns about conventional agriculture. Food is an emotional issue, for good reason. By now consumers have been conditioned to take the "latest report" with a grain of salt and an occasional dash of dread. Headlines extol the health benefits of something one week, then warn of its dangers the next. Shoppers are left holding the grocery bag, unable to sift fact from fiction.

Our intention is to be fair to both sides, and our goal is to help you make intelligent choices about organic food. In so doing, we acknowledge the hard work of the decent, dedicated people—working in both the organic and the conventional food industries—who care deeply about the implications of modern food production.

Because we Americans have been so blessed with a plentiful and inexpensive food supply, we don't often take the time to think about the impact of our food purchases. We make decisions on every trip to the grocery store, but beyond the shelf and behind the labels, there's a story to tell. How our food is produced directly affects the life and health of our culture. It's about you, your family, your community, all of us: shuffling through the aisles, holding options to the light, comparing apples with apples.

We have entered the Organic Age.

So far our ability to reason has made us all foragers for information. Here's to hoping we do well with the fruits of our labor.

Luddene Perry

A Note to the Reader

This is a different kind of buying guide: one that takes you and your values into account, and that allows you the freedom to exercise those values when making choices at the grocery store. We believe that becoming a truly informed organic consumer involves more than gaining a working knowledge of USDA standards. To help you become more informed, we have divided the book into two parts, each playing an integral role in helping you determine which organic food purchases are right for you.

Part I serves as a primer on organic foods, explaining the Organic Foods Production Act and the USDA seals in plain language from the consumer's perspective. It includes examples of the different organic labels you will find in your local supermarket or natural foods store. It also provides background on and outlines the major issues that affect the growing, selling, and regulating of organic food today. Part II leads you through seven grocery aisles, highlighting issues specific to each product group. By applying your broadened understanding, you will more easily recognize the products that best address the issues you care about.

The two parts work together to establish a foundation of knowledge upon which your choices will ultimately rest. To help you determine your current organic shopping habits, we have included a brief survey at the beginning of Part I. At the beginning of Part II, we offer another set of questions that will help you determine the type of organic shopper you want to become.

In short, you are an important part of this book, and the guidance we provide acknowledges your role in deciding for yourself how you wish to express your values at the checkout counter.

PART I
Organic Foods and You

SINCE OUR GOAL is to help you define what buying organic means to you, we have created a brief survey to determine your current understanding of organic food. Each question measures the importance you place on the potential benefits of buying organic.

To complete the survey, check only those responses that apply to you. When you are finished, add up your score. The result will give you some idea about the type of organic food buyer you are right now.

YOUR ORGANIC SHOPPING PROFILE

I search out and purchase organic foods

• more than once a week	4
• weekly	3
• once a month	2
• every few months	1
• never	0

I usually spend my organic dollar on

• dairy	1
• beverages	1
• meat	1
• produce	1
• packaged items	1

Organic foods usually cost more than their conventionally produced equivalents, but I'll buy them if they cost

• the same as conventional items	1
• up to 25% more	1
• up to 50% more	2
• up to 75% more	3
• up to 100% or more	4

I buy organic because I believe it is

• healthier	10
• better for the environment	10
• better for society	10
• all of the above	30
• none of the above	0

Total	__

Now add up your score and determine your Organic Shopping Profile.* If your score was

■ 10–19: you are a *Basic* Organic Shopper. That means you are:

- Just beginning to buy organics
- Not fully convinced of the benefits
- Familiar with a very small number of organic brands
- Primarily concerned with health benefits

---

* This profile is loosely based on studies that place shoppers into different categories depending on the type and frequency of their organic purchases. Although these studies—intended to assist retailers with marketing—offer a more elaborate picture of consumer habits, we have chosen three categories.

■ 20–29: you are a *Choice* Organic Shopper. That means you are:

- Somewhat focused on buying organics
- Expanding the number and type of organic products you purchase
- Convinced that organics have *some* benefits
- Becoming more familiar with organic brands
- Driven by health benefits but are concerned about the environmental impact of growing food as well

■ 30+: you are a *Classic* Organic Shopper. That means you are:

- Very focused on buying organics
- Buying almost exclusively organics
- Eager to learn more about brands and new products
- Convinced of the many benefits that organics provide
- Aware of organics' environmental benefits and social implications

Look at the characteristics of your Organic Shopping Profile. If your answers place you in one but you feel you belong in another, don't give up. Because of the wide range of scores, there will be considerable overlap.

As you read the next chapters, periodically ask yourself if your new knowledge is making you more or less likely to buy organic products. At the beginning of Part II, another self-assessment will offer you an opportunity to further your understanding of both the subjects discussed and your reaction to them.

CHAPTER 1
Organics 101

I T'S EASY TO OVERLOOK the miracle of the modern American supermarket and the complex industry that feeds us. Every week we stroll through brightly lit aisles, surrounded by the least expensive and most abundant food supply in the world, dropping items into a cart without much thought about where it all comes from.[1] Shopping for sustenance is natural to us, and we rarely stop to consider the vast industrial network that allows us this luxury.

Americans' lack of connection to food production is understandable. In 1900 farmers made up 38 percent of the country's workforce.[2] Today that figure is less than 2 percent, and the closest most of us get to a farm is driving past fields at seventy miles per hour.[3] The fact that only a small number of people produce enough food to supply each man, woman, and child in the United States with more than 3,500 calories per day is testament to the incredible efficiency of industrial agriculture. Americans never have to worry about finding store shelves empty. We simply buy what we want and eat it.

Because our system of food distribution separates us from the soil, we experience food as colorful packages bagged in paper or plastic. It's hard to imagine the people, places, and processes that make it all possible. In some cases—our meat supply, for example—we exercise a willful ignorance and would just as soon avoid the grisly, gristly details. We prefer to think about happy cows on milk cartons, playful cereal box tigers, and friendly green giants on cans.

Even when we do allow ourselves a thought about the variety and quantity of food available to us, our curiosity collapses under the weight of production statistics that we cannot readily comprehend—a direct result of the progress made in the last century. Just one hundred years ago—when almost half the population was either growing crops, gathering eggs, or milking cows—the average lifespan in the United States was shorter by twenty-seven years,[4] and a much greater percentage of people died or became ill from food-related problems.

But this progress has exacted considerable costs. The industrialization of agriculture (and of culture in general), while improving our lives in many ways, also separates us from the source of our sustenance—the soil. This disconnect poses problems for our health, our environment, and our society.

THE ORGANIC RESPONSE

How does organic food fit into all this? Simply put, the industrialization of agriculture prompted a response: organic farming. But most American consumers have only recently become aware of organic products, as natural food chains, supermarkets, and even Wal-Mart have introduced this segment of the food industry to a wider audience.

Shopping for groceries today means confronting new choices among goods that appear to be identical except for their prices and the addition of "organic" labels. Based on our notions of organic, we make assumptions about these products, but what do we really know? We may understand that an organic product is grown without synthetic fertilizers, chemical pesticides, growth hormones, or anti-biotics. Beyond that, we are left with several basic questions:

- What exactly does it mean when food is labeled "organic"?
- How do we know the products we buy are organic?
- Where does all this organic food come from?

Here's the short course. In 1990 Congress passed the Organic Foods Production Act (OFPA). Twelve years later, beginning on October 21, 2002, organic food became eligible for official USDA recognition. The "organic" labels and products you find in stores today are the result of this law, and the law itself is the result of a long, flavorful history of ideological struggle and political wrangling.[5] When you buy an organic product, you are paying for an assurance that the product is different—perhaps better—than its conventional counterpart.

The following brief guided tour through the labels will help you understand exactly what this law means to you in the grocery store.

BEHIND THE SEAL

The first thing to remember is that any product now sold in the United States that claims to be "organic" must meet the criteria of the USDA's National Organic Program (NOP), set forth in the OFPA. Although the USDA seal is not required, any organic product must include the name and address of a certifying agency accredited by the USDA.[6] In other words, if it says "organic," it has to meet the government standards, and it will most likely display this seal:

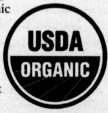

The second thing that the well-informed organic shopper should know is that all organic foods are not created equal. Depending on the percentage of organic ingredients a product contains, it falls into one of four categories— only two of which are eligible for official recognition on the Principal Display Panel (PDP), meaning the front of the jar, can, bag, or box.

We'll use salsa as an example and start with the top of the line. The PDP will look like this:

100% Organic Label

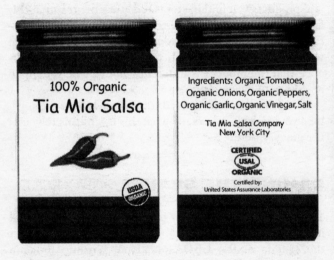

The "organic" label with a percentage included may seem self-explanatory, but remember: whether it's 100 percent organic or just organic, the seal itself will look the same. The difference between the product labeled "organic" and one that includes a percentage is a matter of a few percentage points of ingredients.

With the "100% organic" label, every ingredient in the box, can, or jar must be grown organically, except for the

salt and water (which are not certifiable). As with all food
products sold in the United States, the water must conform to the federal safe drinking water standards. Unlike
conventional products, the salt in organic products cannot
contain a flowing agent.* In addition, none of the ingredients can be irradiated, contain genetically engineered organisms (GEOs), or be grown with sewage sludge fertilizer—the
so-called big three.

Organic Label

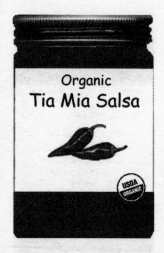
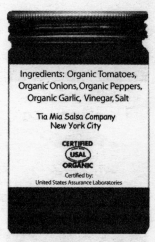

A product labeled "organic" means that at least 95 percent of its ingredients (either by weight or by volume)
must be organic. To meet this criterion is to be as close to
perfect as is vegetably possible. For example, during the
process of making salsa, let's say the supply of organic

---

* The additive that keeps salt from getting lumpy and, incidentally, the
  inspiration for Morton Salt's girl with the umbrella—"When it rains,
  it pours."

vinegar becomes dangerously low and therefore unavailable. A letter is placed on file from the vinegar source stating that it cannot supply the salsa maker with organic vinegar, and conventional vinegar enters the salsa.[7] If the conventional ingredient is not affected by the big three, makes up less than 5 percent of the total ingredients, and is clearly listed in the ingredient panel, the product may be certified "organic."

Made with Organic Label

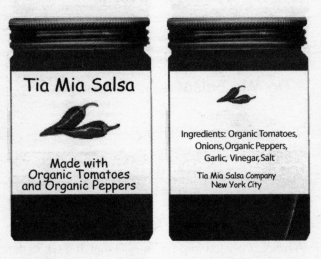

Tia Mia Salsa

Made with
Organic Tomatoes
and Organic Peppers

Ingredients: Organic Tomatoes,
Onions, Organic Peppers,
Garlic, Vinegar, Salt

Tia Mia Salsa Company
New York City

Principal Display Panel   **Ingredient Panel**

The third category of organically labeled foods will be less visible because these products are not allowed to use the word *organic* as a description of the product. Even though it isn't eligible for a USDA seal or a certifier's logo, the product may include the words "made with organic ingredients" and list up to three organic ingredients on the PDP. The "made with . . ." rating requires that at least 70 percent of the ingredients be grown, shipped, and packaged according to organic standards, and the big three rules still apply, even in the remaining 30 percent of nonorganic ingredients.

Less Than 70% Organic Label

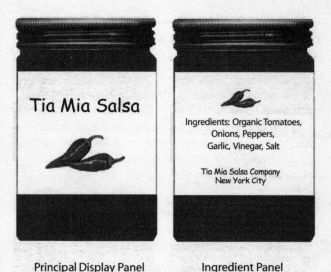

Principal Display Panel   Ingredient Panel

The last type of organic product bears no seal or certifier's logo and contains less than 70 percent organic ingredients. Organic ingredients can be listed on the back panel, but all references to the organic content of the product are prohibited on the PDP in order to "assure that these statements are not displayed in such a manner as to misrepresent the actual organic composition of the product."[8] In this last category, the big three *are allowed* in the nonorganic ingredients. Because it makes little sense for a manufacturer to pay for organic ingredients without being able to advertise them, chances are you won't see many of these products unless organic labeling standards change to meet industry demands.

In addition to the official seal, you may also confront a number of other labels and certifications (see sidebar below and on next page).

TRADITIONAL ORGANIC . . . NATURALLY

"Natural," "organic," "pesticide-free," "traditional": is it any wonder that consumers are confused? What does each label mean, exactly?

For starters, the term *organic* is the only one on the list currently regulated by the U.S. government. The others have no official definition. Here are a few alternative labels and what they mean:

- **Certified organic:** The product has been produced according to the National Organic Program's rule and certified to be in compliance with the rule by an independent, USDA-accredited certifier.

- **Organic, not certified:** Only producers who raise less than $5,000 worth of products per year are eligible to label products "organic" without being certified. They still must play by the rules, and their products cannot be used in foods that are labeled with the USDA seal.

- **Natural:** The product contains no artificial ingredients or added colors and is only minimally processed (in a way that does not fundamentally alter the raw product). The label must explain the use of the term *natural* (such as "no added colorings or artificial ingredients").

- **Traditional:** While evoking green pastures and happy farm families, the term is unregulated.

- **Free-range:** Usually applied to poultry, this term means any livestock raised with unlimited access to the outdoors.

- **Pastured:** This term is similar to *free-range,* but with emphasis on "managed pasture." Such pastures are maintained by rotating the animals to prevent the forage from being overgrazed. Any livestock—chickens, hogs, sheep, and the like—can be pasture-raised. If no other supplement feed has been given, then *pastured* can turn into *grass-fed.*

- **Grass-fed:** Grass-fed animals (usually cattle or milk cows) are those that eat only what they were designed to eat: grasses. Organic regulations do not require grass-feeding exclusively.

- **Biodynamic:** Biodynamics is an organic production method that adheres to the tenets of Rudolf Steiner. All biodynamic crops are also organic, but the NOP disqualifies the term *biodynamic.* To attain USDA certification, the biodynamic movement developed a certifying agency named Stellar—with different standards—to qualify for accreditation by the USDA.

- **Other eco-labels:** The Consumers Union offers a wonderful online resource to assist shoppers with the ever-increasing number of new labels and certifications at www.eco-labels.org/home.cfm.

BEFORE THE SEAL: THE CERTIFICATION PROCESS

The law that governs organic foods is a labeling law, but the seal on the package forms the epilogue of a story that begins at least three years before you buy a product. That's how long a farm must be free of chemical pesticides and fertilizers before it can be certified. And there's a lot more to it than that. The standards regulate the whole chain of events from the farm to the supermarket shelf.

So how do you know that what you buy is actually organic? An independent third party—a certifying agency—spends considerable time and effort to guarantee that the product meets the following criteria:

- Three years before a farmer can sell any organic crops, he or she applies for certification from an agency accredited by the USDA. Some applications can be one hundred pages long, and the requested information may take the farmer weeks or months to compile.

- These applications often serve as the USDA's mandated "organic plan." This plan acts as the blueprint for maintaining the organic integrity of the farm.

- The certifying agency then reviews the plan with a paid staff or volunteer committee. If the certifying agency is satisfied that the farmer understands and is committed to the principles of organic farming, it calls for an independent inspection. Most inspectors are not directly employed by the agency, and are members of the Independent Organic Inspectors Association (IOIA). Yearly inspections are required for both farms and processing facilities.

- All aspects of the farm—pest control, buildings, equipment, and crop rotations—must be documented by the farmer, confirmed by the inspector, and accepted by the agency.

- Each field must be mapped and have a detailed field activity log (essentially, a dated record of everything the farmer does in that field).

- When the inspection forms are finally submitted, the review committee then studies them in detail and decides whether to grant certification.

The above steps refer to farming operations, but food-processing facilities are held to the same scrutiny. A certifier inspects every inch of the plant, from the delivery dock to the file cabinet in the office. It may take over a year to certify a processing facility that manufactures multi-ingredient products, because each product must be documented and an audit trail established. The certifying agency will insist that an inspector verify each of these documents for *every* ingredient. When an agency has acquired all of the documentation and is confident the applicant is compliant, it then grants certification.

WHAT IS AN AUDIT TRAIL?

Every organic product can be traced to the field in which it was grown with a series of documents known as an *audit trail.* This trail provides proof that a given food producer or processor is playing by the rules. When a company or grower has met all the criteria, it receives a certificate, which should be available to consumers upon request. The certificate, however, is just one document in an audit trail. Others include: field histories; production activity records; farm input records; harvest records; storage records; weigh tickets; farmer's organic certificates; bills of lading; clean truck affidavits; inventory purchase records; production reports; packaging reports; finished product reports;

shipping reports; maintenance and sanitation records; a list of ingredient suppliers; pesticide management records; product formulations; "big three" affidavits (GEOs, irradiation, sewage sludge); sales invoices of the final product; and an audit control register.

The certifying agency will insist on complete transparency, acting as the consumer's eyes and ears. It may seem tedious, but this tightly controlled process ultimately leads to the organic seal you see in the supermarket. The certifying agency's approval becomes your only source of information about the validity of the organic products you buy. If you have questions about how a particular organic product achieved certification, you should be able to contact the certifying agency whose name and contact information appear on the package. However, our own attempts to do so have been less than successful as the certifying industry grows.

CERTIFYING AGENCIES

Crop certification dates back to at least the 1890s, when crop improvement associations (CIAs) formed to guarantee farmers that the seeds they planted were true to type. In the 1970s early organic certifiers adopted many of the methods and procedures pioneered by CIAs. During this time, there were only a few organic certifiers, and they struggled through inadequate funds and turf wars. Some organic advocates trace the development of the Organic Food Production Act directly to the conflicts among certifying groups.

With OFPA's passage in 1990, several groups and individuals saw potential profit in certification, and the number of certifiers grew to about thirty by 1992. These certification agents took one of three forms: nonprofit associations, state agriculture departments, and private (for-profit) companies. As the implementation date neared, the number of groups grew, and by August 2004 the NOP's website listed fifty-eight accredited domestic certifiers, sixteen of which were state or county government agencies. An additional thirty-seven foreign certifiers were also listed.

The number of new certifiers has triggered concerns among some in the organic community—particularly the inclusion of for-profit agencies. Certification, they said, was very exacting. Did these new certifiers have the experience to do the job correctly? Would the profit motive lead to shoddy and inadequate certifications?

Despite the large number of certifiers, consumers will most likely see only one of about four or five certification seals on products, because the majority of agencies certify farms. Only a few specialize in certifying the packaged products you find at the store. One for-profit agency, Quality Assurance International (QAI), now certifies 70 to 80 percent of all organic packaged products. Moreover, this agency has been bought by a larger commercial interest with no connection to the organic industry, prompting raised eyebrows among advocates concerned about the "selling out" of organic integrity.

THE PRICE OF ORGANICS

For most consumers, the higher price of organic food is the primary impediment to purchase. While advocates agree that organic foods cost more, they see the extra expense as a more accurate reflection of the real cost of food grown in a truly sustainable system. Critics counter that organics' higher prices are little more than a marketing gimmick and that organic foods represent an elitist luxury in what is fast becoming a two-tiered, class-based food system. Both sides make valid points that really go hand in hand.

Organic agriculture's additional requirements do add to the end cost, but so does the limited supply of organic foods. Building large acreages of nutrient-rich soil without the use of chemicals means that producers must develop yield-reducing crop-rotation schemes or must buy and transport less efficient natural nutrient inputs like manure, chicken feather compost, or bat guano. While chemical-free production methods have obvious benefits, they have yet to *consistently* match conventional yields on a large scale.

Production methods alone do not determine price. Different retail outlets serve different needs in the organic food–buying community. National chains like Whole Foods Markets offer an alternative grocery-shopping experience designed to make consumers feel healthy, wealthy, and wise. These stores have an upscale feel, but with their larger inventories, national chains are very competitive, and in our experience, organic foods purchased there are cheaper than organic foods purchased at our local conventional supermarket.*

Co-ops generally offer a more proletarian feel without elaborate displays, gourmet coffee shops, or juice bars, although some are now following the large-chain lead. For the most part, however, they offer fresh produce and other organic goods in smaller displays, devoting more space to bulk bins. Most shoppers *perceive* co-ops as being less

---

* This may not be true of Wal-Mart, which is now one of the nation's leading organic food retailers and always seems to find a way to roll back prices.

expensive than chains or conventional supermarkets, but this was not necessarily our experience.

The following price comparison was taken the week of May 14, 2004. All prices compared were the same brand and size.

	Supermarket		Whole Foods Market	Food Co-op
ITEM	Conventional	Organic	Organic	Organic
Apples, 1#	$0.67	$0.75	$1.99	$1.59
Carrots, 2#	$1.22	$1.99	$1.99	$1.49
Frzn. strawberries, 10 oz.	$2.59	$3.99	$3.99	$3.99
2% milk, 1/2 gal.	$2.39	$2.99	$3.49	$3.09
Silk Soymilk, 1/2 gal.	$2.99	$2.99	$2.99	$3.29
Large eggs, 1 doz.	$1.10	$3.69	$3.39	$3.29
Butter, 1#	$2.99	$5.69	$4.79	$5.29
Vanilla yogurt, 6 oz.	$0.99	$1.09	$0.89	$0.99
Whole wheat bread	$2.69	$3.59	$3.19	$3.29
Cereal	$3.19	$4.49	$3.99	$4.29
Canned pinto beans	$0.69	$1.59	$1.39	$1.39
Peanut butter	$1.86	$4.79	$3.75	$3.99
Ketchup	$1.39	$1.99	$1.99	$3.49
Mac & cheese	$0.79	$2.15	$1.79	$1.59
Frozen vegetable lasagna	$2.25	$4.19	$3.69	$4.19
Apple juice	$1.38	$3.79	$2.89	$2.14
Chai	$2.79	$3.69	$3.29	$4.59
Cream-filled cookies	$3.19	$3.49	$3.39	$3.69
Corn chips	$2.29	$2.79	$3.29	$3.69
Total	$38.64	$60.73	$56.77	$52.44*

* Without member discount

MORE THAN ATMOSPHERE

Although buying organic items at your local supermarket may be a more convenient proposition, the truly health-conscious shopper may want to seek out a market that has been certified organic or at the very least displays a GORP sign. GORP (Good Retail Organic Practices) is a program developed by the Organic Trade Association to train store personnel in proper handling, storage, and packaging of organic food. A significant portion of the training involves handling various aspects of retail pest control.

Most conventional supermarkets routinely spray for cockroaches, ants, and other undesirables. To control rodents, bait stations containing potent anticoagulants are placed along the outside of the building, and "tin cat" mousetraps line the walls of storage areas. All of these control measures may contribute to the possibility of contamination if they are not handled with care.

Then there's the issue of packaging. In the days when food co-ops were just getting started, few people understood the dangers of using unapproved food containers. I worked in food co-ops that employed all manner of boxes and plastic containers to store and display food. Today we know that plastic "leaks" chemicals, and that boxes are frequently permeated with pesticides. Only GORP-trained workers know all the ins and outs of proper handling techniques.

ACCOUNTING FOR TASTE

Given the higher prices and more stringent production methods, some consumers naturally assume that organic foods taste better. Indeed, pro-organic books and websites insist that it does. The problem with these kinds of pronouncements is their vagueness. Exactly what types of organic foods taste better? On what do they base their assertions?

In general, fresh produce gets the taste-test attention, although little "scientific" data exists on the subject—as it should be, given that taste is highly subjective. Furthermore, food is not like other testable products, in that so many factors—weather, soil conditions, and handling, to name a few—influence a food product's taste. Nevertheless, formal and informal studies have been done. One such study conducted at Washington State University found organic apples tasted sweeter than conventional apples. Whether sweeter apples are better is, of course, a personal matter.

We have conducted both blind and open informal taste tests on fruits and vegetables, bread, cereal, peanut butter, cheese, eggs, chicken, steak, juice, cookies, and frozen entrees. You will find these "taste checks" throughout the Aisle chapters. With some products, we compared organic not just with conventional supermarket items but with nonorganic locally produced fare. Results were never conclusive, except that the freshest, least processed products always tasted better to us. In short, any produce fresh from the garden is going to beat the pants off any vegetable packaged in plastic and shipped thousands of miles.

Another thing to keep in mind when talking about taste is the variety. There is no contest between the flavor of an heirloom Brandywine tomato and a commercially bred UG 606 tomato from United Genetics. Whereas large organic producers mimic the packing, processing, and shipping requirements of large conventional producers, many small organic growers choose especially succulent varieties over those bred for shipping qualities, processing characteristics, or disease resistance. If you want better-tasting produce, seek local growers who offer different varieties whether they are certified organic or not—which leads to another reason why some organic food may taste better.

In general, companies inclined to become organic began their lives as small operations with a tradition of making fine products with limited distribution. For instance, I've tasted organic white cheddar made by Cedar Grove Cheese Factory in Plain, Wisconsin. I've also had their conventional white cheddar. Both were exceptionally good. Taste isn't necessarily about being organic. It's about the producer taking the time to make a quality product.

Finally, we watched with interest when someone from CBS's program *Sunday Morning* stood on a Manhattan sidewalk and offered organic and conventional strawberries to pedestrians. While the test was blind, it was not exactly scientific, but it confirmed our own findings. Some thought the organic tasted better. Others opted for the conventional. But it still didn't answer the real question at the heart of the issue: Does how we treat the soil make a difference in how food tastes? To design a truly valid taste test, researchers would have to grow the same variety of vegetable or fruit in the same climate at the same time in the same soil. The only difference would be in the production method itself. Such tests have not been widely conducted.

If you believe organic foods taste better, words are not going to change your mind, and we decided early on that in this book we were not going to attempt to be arbiters of taste. Ultimately, only you can answer this question on a week-by-week basis.

DECISIONS, DECISIONS

Back at the wall of salsa, with an organic jar in your left hand and a conventional jar in your right, you compare prices and wonder if organic salsa will better complement the tortilla chips and guacamole already captive in the cage of your cart. Is the item you hold worth the extra money?

Advocates make a number of claims about organic food's superiority: it has more nutrients, tastes better, and is safer to eat. It protects wildlife, water, and soil. It saves family farms and enhances farm workers' well-being. Are these claims accurate?

Answering these questions is not easy and largely depends on possessing some background knowledge about the health, environmental, and societal issues addressed by organic food. In the next four chapters we'll explore the history and evolution of organic production methods and the concerns they seek to address.

CHAPTER 2

The Evolution of Organic Agriculture

FROM THE SHOPPER'S PERSPECTIVE in the supermarket aisle, the promise of organic food seems straightforward enough. If the criteria are met, the end product gets the government's plainspoken seal—a field of green (or black) 'neath a white USDA sky. But the seal's simplicity belies the rich history of ideas and impassioned struggles to define the principles and practices of organic agriculture. For those involved in the production of organic food, and for a growing number of savvy consumers, the government's stamp of approval is not the be-all and end-all of what it means to be organic.

DEFINING *ORGANICS*

As you come to understand what organics means to you, it might be helpful to think of the USDA regulations as a mark on a continuum of agricultural practices, with conventional practices on the right and "beyond organic" practices to the left. Where you fall on this continuum represents your specific values, and the food-buying choices you make will reflect those values.

As you expand your knowledge of food-production practices, many of you will decide that the current USDA standards suffice. Some of you—after careful consideration of the issues involved—will seek out alternatives that more precisely meet your expectations. And some of you may decide that conventional food standards—when all is said and done—meet your needs just fine.

Whatever your conclusions, a basic understanding of the organic agricultural debate is a good place to start.

THE LAY OF THE LAND

If you are new to organics, you may be surprised to learn that there is considerable controversy within the organic movement about the direction of the industry. In general, this debate pits committed idealism against the realities of commerce. To get a deeper grasp of this issue, compare the views of Fred Kirschenmann, a longtime organic farmer, with those of Gene Kahn, founder of Cascadian Farms. Both men present compelling arguments in the struggle to shape organic agriculture today and in the future.

Organic advocate Joan Dye Gussow once asked a now-famous question: *Can an organic Twinkie be certified?* In the simplest terms, how you answer it offers a glimpse into the type of organic shopper you want to be. For those in the Kirschenmann camp, the specter of an organic Twinkie—a symbol for the highly processed products of industrial food production—casts a pall over the future of organics. For those who side with Gene Kahn, the future of organics rests on the ability of organic producers to offer consumers a wider array of processed products.

Aside from the internal debate, organic agriculture has its vocal detractors as well. Criticism usually takes one of two forms: the practical and the cultural. Practical critics decry organics' disdain for what they see as essential technological developments—synthetic pesticides and fertilizers being the most obvious. They insist that truly organic methods are unworkable on a large scale. Cultural critics, for their part, attack organics for being a marketing gimmick that caters to the wealthy.

As you define and refine your feelings about organic agriculture, a little history always helps to flesh out opinion. Organics did not just emerge fully formed when the USDA seal appeared on products. Organics today must be placed in the context of food production in the last hundred years.

ORGANICS IN CONTEXT

The first few decades of the twentieth century ushered in enormous changes in the way food was grown and processed. In the fields, manufactured fertilizers replaced traditional methods of enriching the soil with animal and plant waste; tractors took the horse out of horsepower; and the time-honored craft of agriculture became an industrial process. Advances in nutrition studies and the discovery of vitamins gave credence to the role of science in food processing. Pioneers such as J. Harvey Kellogg (packaged cereal) and Charles Birdseye (frozen foods) popularized factory-made foodstuffs. At the time, the majority of the American public reacted positively, swept up by the cleanliness and convenience of modern methods.

But not everyone shared the enthusiasm for food grown with chemicals or cooked up in laboratories. For some, the intrusion of science into the sacred territory of sustenance signaled the decline—not the advancement—of civilization. Food processing stripped away vital nutrients, and the symbol of processing—refined white flour—became one of the disagreements *du jour*.[1] While industrialists saw it as clean and pure, the "proto-organicists" deemed it artificial and unhealthy. In many ways, flour epitomized the later debate about conventional versus organic methods:

the struggle between a resolute trust in science and a desire to return to a more "natural" past.

Born in the Soil

Because the present-day organic movement emerged from the mists of an agricultural past thrust into modernity, we cannot point directly to a single event as the genesis. Some advocates claim organics began in the 1940s with J. I. Rodale. Others cite Lady Eve Balfour and Sir Albert Howard's contributions in the 1930s. Still others trace organics' roots to Germany in the late 1800s, when philosophers and idealists eventually coalesced in the *Naturmenschen* (natural men) and the *Lebensreform* (life-reform) movements. Many of those involved in these movements immigrated to California, where they sought to live a natural life in the Sunshine State. From 1915 until the late 1940s, these seekers pioneered many aspects of California's health food movement, which later formed the backbone of the natural food movement in the 1960s and 1970s—an important component in the spread of organics.

If we take as its starting point the term *organic*, Sir Albert Howard laid the groundwork. From 1905 to 1931, Howard studied compost heaps in India for the British government. His work there focused on advancing inexpensive and innovative soil-building techniques using natural processes—a much different approach from that taken by soil chemists, whose work led to the development of synthetic fertilizers.

Howard believed that "artificial fertilizers lead to artificial nutrition, artificial animals, and finally to artificial men and women."[2] By focusing on the microbes feasting on decayed vegetable matter, he speculated that the essential

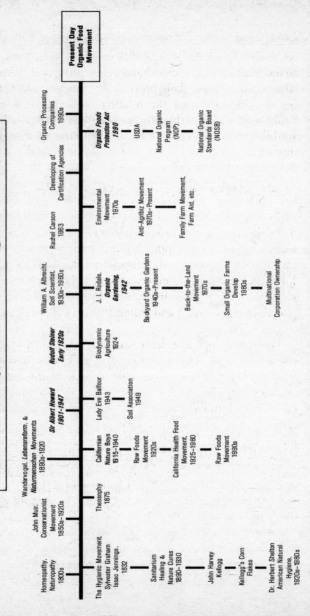

Historical Components of the Organic Movement

Present Day Organic Food Movement

Organic Processing Companies
1990s

Organic Foods Protection Act 1990
USDA
National Organic Program (NOP)
National Organic Standards Board (NOSB)

Developing of Certification Agencies

Rachel Carson 1983
Environmental Movement 1970s
Anti-Agribiz Movement 1970s–Present
Family Farm Movement, Farm Aid, etc.

William A. Albrecht, Soil Scientist, 1930s–1960s
J. I. Rodale, *Organic Gardening*, 1942
Backyard Organic Gardens 1940s–Present
Back-to-the-Land Movement 1970s
Small Organic Farms Develop 1980s
Multinational Corporation Ownership

Rudolf Steiner Early 1920s
Biodynamic Agriculture 1924

Sir Albert Howard 1901–1947
Lady Eve Balfour 1943
Soil Association 1949

Wandervogel, *Lebensreform* & *Naturmenschen* Movements 1890s–1920

John Muir, Conservationist Movement 1850s–1920s
Theosophy 1875
Californian Nature Boys 1915–1940
Raw Foods Movement 1920s
California Health Food Movement, 1925–1960
Raw Foods Movement 1990s

Homeopathy, Naturopathy, 1800s
The Hygienic Movement Sylvester Graham Issac Jennings, 1832
Sanitarium Healing & Nature Cures 1890–1930
John Harvey Kellogg
Kellogg's Corn Flakes
Dr. Herbert Shelton American Natural Hygiene, 1920s–1980s

organic matter (humus) resulting from compost supplied a "unique essence" for growth. He connected deficient soil to the human health "crisis" and called industrial methods "the murder of our daily bread."[3] Although he supported his conclusions about the relationship between human health and soil health with anecdotal evidence, his soil studies are regarded as influential within the organic community.

Healthy Soil, Healthy People

In the United States, Howard's theories inspired a former IRS accountant to seek a more healthful lifestyle.[4] Concerned about the industrialization of the food supply, and driven by the notion that organic matter was the answer, J. I. Rodale moved his family to a farm in Pennsylvania. He succeeded in restoring its fertility through the liberal application of compost[5] and called this production method "organic."[6]

For Rodale, organic food was about health and a respect for nature. His definition of *organic* was "a system whereby a fertile soil is maintained by applying nature's own law of replenishing it—that is, the addition and preservation of humus, the use of organic matter instead of chemical fertilizers, and of course the making of a compost pile."[7] Despite all the debate about what *organic* means today, the betterment of human health through compost was the recipe for the early organic movement. While additional ingredients would later be added, Howard's and Rodale's ideas initially formed the core of organic philosophy.

From Health to a Healthier Environment

Rodale was not alone in pointing out industrial agriculture's shortcomings. While he (and others in the U.K., Germany, and Japan) associated industrial methods with poor human health, Rachel Carson took it one step further. Carson wrote *Silent Spring* in 1962, and its publication opened a floodgate of concern over chemicals awash in our daily lives. In the year following its publication, Carson testified before Congress while she herself was dying of breast cancer. Her book and subsequent testimony charged that industrial chemicals—particularly pesticides—were responsible for creating a cancer epidemic and decimating wildlife.

Although many of Carson's claims about pesticides and cancer have long been the subject of debate, her forceful, poetic arguments helped inspire a fledgling environmental movement. Activists targeted every chemical substance, manufacturing process, and agricultural technique that could possibly be linked to environmental degradation. Neither the food-processing industry nor the agricultural community went unexamined. The pejorative term *agribiz* was coined to refer to profit-hungry corporations that seemed oblivious to the debasement of the food supply and the environment. A new generation of organic growers and natural food seekers found common cause with aging organic practitioners who subscribed to Rodale's magazine. After *Silent Spring,* organic advocates made pesticides and the environment their central concern. For them, organics offered a solution to agricultural pollution.

Adapting to its time, the Rodale Press began promoting a connection between organic agriculture and the environmental movement. Its magazines and books presented the idea that if farmers would give up conventional practices and convert to organic, they could control soil erosion, reduce groundwater contamination, and prevent further decline in biodiversity. In response, young, starry-eyed organic warriors took up the call and poured out of the cities in the great "back to the land" movement.

Most of these new, organic hopefuls assumed that the prevailing principle of organic farming was the elimination of chemicals. When the realization struck that organic agriculture is more than chemical-free farming, a number of neophyte farmers fled back to their urban havens. Few had grasped the enormous effort required for sound soil-building techniques. But some small farms did succeed by producing food organically and selling it through a network of food co-ops. Some triumphed with organics, while others moved into sustainable agriculture, eco-agriculture, or biodynamics. Eventually each of these methods found a niche, and some turned into thriving businesses that later formed the core of the organic community.

Ever alert to the possibility of new markets, the conventional food industry saw an opportunity in the "natural foods" counterculture. Yogurt and whole-wheat bread captured the zeitgeist, and granola remains emblematic of its time, but these foods changed considerably in the hands of large food companies. Sugar was added to yogurt, while extra fat and sweeteners found their way into granola. The industry's incorporation of natural foods into their product lines was a harbinger of things to come: large food companies have now adopted organic production methods to manufacture highly processed, packaged goods.

Running parallel to the food industry's co-optation of natural foods, the organic movement continued to grow, expanding its list of health concerns and environmental issues associated with industrial agriculture.

From Environmental Health to Societal Health

Concerns about industrial agriculture's impact on the environment led to further scrutiny of its failings in other areas. Often described as "social justice" issues, these problems cover a number of diverse areas related to corporate control over the production, processing, and distribution of the food supply. One example is the rise of "factory farming," which accompanied the decline of the small farmer. By the time the Farm Aid concerts began in 1985, advocates saw organics as one of the few remaining hopes for saving the family farm and protecting the well-being of farm workers.

While many within the movement saw a need to add a social component to organic standards, they did not become part of the law in the United States. But inclusion of social justice standards in the international organic community is currently under way.

Organics Today

In order to meet the growing demand for organic food, modern organic production methods have adopted some of the trappings of industrial agriculture. Many of the original organic growers are now part of the same global "agribiz" machine that the early organic movement saw as the source of the problem. This is not to say that multinational corporations (and the smaller organic companies they have an interest in) are not following the standards and doing good things, but as organics becomes a more sophisticated industry, questions about what *organic* means will continue to emerge. The laws of supply and demand have created a dilemma for the organic movement.

ORGANIC THINKING

The organic industry today must confront a problem similar to that faced by agriculture as it became industrialized: how to supply the market's demands. The conventional solution involves methods and practices that are deemed unacceptable to the organic way of thinking. To the organically inclined, progress is not a headlong rush into the unknown but a slow development, respectful of the natural world and our place in it. While growing crops and domesticating animals necessitates an alteration of the environment, the practices of *industrial* agriculture—monocropping, overcrowded feedlots, and synthetic inputs—are especially harmful to the environment and to us.

Given this philosophical background, it is not surprising that organic advocates see conventional agriculture as a system driven by profits over people.

ASSESSING ORGANICS

As you define your own organic ethic, the relative worth of organics depends on your assessment of the differences between organic and conventional agriculture. But simply comparing one production method with another, then weighing the advantages and disadvantages, is only part of the organic story. The fact that organics have been—and for many, still are—more than a set of production rules both complicates and enriches their value.

Examples of this complexity can be found in Sylvia Tawse's list of ten reasons for buying organic foods. Originally appearing in an article for *Organic Times* in the spring of 1992, it has been adapted and used extensively as a marketing tool for both Whole Foods Markets and the Organic Trade Association. The list, in its many incarnations, was used on shopping bags and remains—in various forms—on hundreds of websites. It appropriately illustrates a wider range of concerns than those addressed by the Organic Foods Production Act:

1. **Protect future generations.** Children receive four times more exposure than adults to cancer-causing pesticides in food.

2. **Prevent soil erosion.** Three billion tons of topsoil are eroded from croplands in the U.S. each year, much of it due to conventional farming practices, which often ignore the health of the soil.

3. **Protect water quality.** The EPA estimates that pesticides pollute the primary source of drinking water for more than half the country's population.

4. **Keep chemicals off your plate.** Pesticides are poisons designed to kill living organisms, and can also be harmful to humans.

5. **Protect farm worker health.** Pesticides are poisons designed to kill living organisms, and can also be harmful to humans.

6. **Save energy.** More energy is now used to produce synthetic fertilizers than to till, cultivate, and harvest all crops in the U.S.

7. **Help small farmers.** Although more and more large scale farms are making the conversion to organic practices, most organic farms are small, independently owned and operated family farms.

8. **Support a true economy.** Organic foods might seem expensive; however, your tax dollars pay for hazardous waste clean-up and environmental damage caused by conventional farming.

9. **Promote biodiversity.** Planting large plots of land with the same crop year after year tripled farm production between 1950 and 1970, but the lack of natural diversity of plant life has negatively affected soil quality.

10. **Flavor and nourishment.** Organic farming starts with the nourishment of the soil, producing nourished, and nourishing, plants. Conduct your own taste test!

Each principle on the list fits into one of three categories that represent the full range of reasons people have for buying organic:

- Organics and health (1, 4, 10)
- Organics and the environment (2, 3, 6, 9)
- Organics and society (5, 7, 8)

In the next three chapters, we will look at each of these three categories in detail.

CHAPTER 3
Organic Foods and Your Health

OF ALL THE CRITICISMS leveled at modern food production, threats to health get the most attention. While industrial agriculture's environmental and social problems can be put on the back burner of our daily lives, health matters get us right where we live. Seventy-four percent of organic food buyers cite health benefits as the primary reason for their purchases.[1] Among these benefits, the belief that organic food is pesticide-free tops the list.

In addition to pesticides, organic proponents mention a number of potential risks with conventional food. The most prevalent are:

- Pesticides
- Antibiotics
- Food additives
- Hormones
- Genetically engineered organisms (GEOs)
- Irradiation
- Nutritional quality
- Mycotoxins
- Pathogens

HEALTH CONCERNS IN CONTEXT

Assessing food-related health risks is an enormously complex endeavor. Understating the potential dangers leaves one open to charges of callousness or industry co-optation while overstating the case for problems with conventional food often creates needless fear in the public mind.

Indeed, Luddene's own pursuit of organics has been inspired by more than thirty years of exposure to criticisms of the conventional food industry. In that time, she accepted at face value the rhetorical and statistical flourishes employed by organic advocates, and dismissed conventional thinking as agribiz propaganda. In retrospect, appealing to consumer fears about health was the only way for the early organic movement—which held little economic or political power—to confront the monolithic conventional food industry. The health benefits touted by the organic industry constitute a sound marketing strategy, but the USDA's seal "is not, at least officially, a health, nutrition or food-safety claim."[2]

Unfortunately, the marketing of health concerns has left organics open to charges of being "unscientific" (see sidebar). While each side preaches to its respective choir, any chance at productive dialogue has become a war of myths and realities: one side's reality is the other's myth, and vice versa.

PESTICIDES

Pesticides embody the paradox of living in an industrial society: we both fear and depend on chemicals. On both counts, it's easy to see why. After all, pesticides are designed to kill living things; yet most people do not want beetles in their flour or cockroaches in their kitchens.

Are Pesticides Necessary?

Recorded in ancient texts such as the *Egyptian Book of the Dead*, the *Odyssey*, and the Bible, the battle against agricultural pests predates the age of chemical corporations by thousands of years.[3] The fact that other living things also like the food we grow and store is indisputable and makes some pest-control measures necessary.[4] The question of pesticides is a matter of the kind of chemicals used, the degree to which they are employed, and the steps that may be taken to alleviate our dependence on them. Organic advocates claim that pest problems are the result of industrial methods of production, such as thousands of acres planted to a single crop. Conventional farmers consider pesticides to be "crop-protection materials" used to ensure a profitable yield.

BILLIONS AND BILLIONS

Man-made chemicals naturally invite some level of suspicion. Adding to those fears are the very large numbers often cited to show how destructive industrial agriculture seems to be. Take this passage from *The Fatal Harvest Reader*:

> Since the mid-1960s, pesticide use on farms has doubled, with nearly a billion pounds of active ingredients now being applied each year. Another 4 billion pounds of "inert" chemicals are added to the pesticide mix, too, including known cancer causers and other toxics. This total pesticide dosage of almost 5 billion pounds a year is 20 pounds for every man, woman, and child in America.

Reading this, you might get the impression that you are being "dosed" with twenty pounds of pesticides (actually four pounds of active ingredient) on your food each year. A closer look at the data reveals a different picture.[5] In fact, herbicides make up the bulk of total agricultural use, and of the pesticides that show up in 2 percent or more of the FDA's Total Diet Study samples, only one is a herbicide (technically, a growth regulator to keep potatoes from sprouting). Why do so few herbicides show up on food? Because these chemicals are used to treat the soil, not the crops themselves. Add to that the nematicides and fumigants (none of which are found on 2 percent of FDA samples), and the amount of pesticides found in table-ready food products goes down considerably.

The idea that you are somehow eating twenty pounds of pesticides is rhetorical sleight-of-hand.

Organic advocates often leave the impression that organic farming eliminates the need for pesticides, insisting that "no one has ever proven that pesticides are necessary to the food supply."[6] If that were true, the Organic Materials Review Institute (OMRI) would have no need to list more than forty pesticides allowed in organic production.[7]

Chemicals on Your Plate

Do pesticide residues show up on food? The easy answer is yes—on some foods some of the time. We know this because the USDA, the FDA, and many states routinely screen for them using highly sensitive tests.

In the popular mind, concerns about pesticide residues tend to center on certain fruits and vegetables, but the bulk of both conventional and organic production is commodity crops: wheat, corn, soybeans, and rice.[8] An examination of the FDA's Total Diet Study reveals that U.S.

commodity crops, when compared to produce, have relatively low rates of residues, so *if you only buy organic because you fear pesticide residues*, products made from grains may be a place to trim your organic food bill. Consumers who have particular concerns about environmental contamination or farm worker health may feel differently.

Health Risks from Residues

When it comes to residues and health, how much is too much? Does your exposure to small amounts of pesticide residues in food pose enough of a risk to pay higher prices?

According to the FDA, residues found on table-ready food range from 0.0001 to 2.04 parts per million (ppm).[9] As a reference point, 1 ppm is the equivalent of one drop in twenty-two gallons, or a grain of salt in a piece of spaghetti as tall as the Empire State Building. The question is whether these small amounts can harm us.

In general, organic advocates say they do and cite a number of possible ills associated with pesticides. Conventional proponents adhere to the toxicology maxim "the dose makes the poison" and insist that current safety standards more than adequately protect consumers.

Are Children More at Risk?

In 1993 the National Research Council looked at the issue of children's special susceptibility to pesticide residues. The report, *Pesticides in the Diets of Infants and Children,* identified some specific risk factors:

- Children tend to eat fewer foods and consequently may be ingesting more of the pesticides found on those foods.
- Children eat more food than adults compared to the size of their bodies.

- Even small amounts of pesticides may disrupt the endocrine and nervous systems at crucial points of development.
- The combined effects of pesticides on food with other household chemicals and drinking water impurities may increase the total toxic load for children.

Three years after the NRC released its report, Congress passed the Food Quality Protection Act (FQPA). The act "set a new standard of a 'reasonable certainty' of no harm that prohibits economic consideration when children are at risk."[10] This means that the EPA sets a standard based on the lowest amount of a chemical that creates observable effects in test animals and automatically decreases the allowable level by a factor of ten. If the chemicals are used in food production, that factor is reduced by another factor of ten. On foods most often eaten by children, the EPA adds an additional margin of safety (another factor of ten) to allowable levels of residues. In addition, FQPA set the EPA on an ambitious reevaluation of currently registered pesticides, curtailing the use of a certain class of pesticides (organophosphates) linked with cancer in children.[11]

These are meaningful reforms and tough new standards, but the EPA hasn't finished reevaluating all currently registered pesticides, so in effect the FQPA has yet to be fully implemented. While you can be reasonably assured that the conventional foods your children have been eating are safe, organic foods offer even better odds— especially if your children tend to eat many of the same types of foods.

The Environmental Estrogen Hypothesis

For most of the last three decades, the study of contaminants in food focused on cancer-causing chemicals and additives, but new concerns about the effects of pesticides on children led to the environmental estrogen hypothesis, or "endocrine disruption theory." The theory proposes that certain chemicals can fool hormone receptors by mimicking estrogen.* This hormonal trickery can trigger reactions that may disrupt growth and development. So far, scientists have not been able to conclusively prove any effect on humans, but evidence—both in the wild and in the laboratory—suggests that even low levels of these chemicals hamper normal sexual development and decrease fertility in fish, birds, and reptiles.

In humans, speculation about other potential health problems related to endocrine disruption includes breast cancer, prostate cancer, immune system dysfunctions, low sperm counts, short penises, and brain irregularities, just to name a few. Again, these effects have not been documented in humans, but for those who support the theory, the "preponderance of evidence"† is enough to merit continued research and concern.

---

* Endocrine-disrupting chemicals include many industrial products. Some are pesticides. Of the pesticides included on the list of known, probable, or suspected "chemicals associated with endocrine system effects in vitro," several are no longer in use. Others, such as atrazine, remain in wide use.

† "Preponderance of evidence" and "weight of evidence" are phrases associated with the Precautionary Principle, which essentially means that if a substance is not *known* to be safe, it should not be used.

Living Through Chemistry

The effects of low-level residues on human health are, at this time, unknown,[12] so we will not repeat the "pesticide residues cause cancer and disrupt hormones" mantra. Nor will we dismiss concerns with a casual "pesticide residues won't hurt you." Like many aspects of modern society, you must weigh the risks against the benefits or costs. For example, should you wear respiratory protection when you pump gas? Maybe. Are the asbestos fibers from brake pads floating in the air at every street corner something to worry about? Possibly.

Avoiding potential hazards with reasonable remedies is obviously a good strategy. Reducing your contact with pesticide residues by buying organic foods may play a role in your personal harm-reduction program. Tests on organic foods tend to show a lower frequency of synthetic pesticide residues,[13] but buying organic food does not guarantee chemical-free food.

ANTIBIOTICS

When these wonder drugs came into wide use, it looked as if modern medicine had made infectious disease a thing of the past. What vaccines did not prevent, antibiotics—our little magic potions—could treat. Today Americans leave their doctors' offices with a prescription 60 percent of the time, often for an antibiotic. In fact, we like them so much we started giving them to livestock. And not just when they were sick—farmers use antibiotics to keep animals healthy and speed their growth. They have become a cure-all for animal production, leaving organic proponents feeling a bit under the weather. Consumers are left to wonder if the antibiotics used in conventional meat and dairy production might cause them harm in the form of residues on food and in the development of antibiotic-resistant bacteria.

In response to concerns about antibiotics, NOP rules do not allow their use. When organically raised animals get sick, they may be treated with "veterinary biologics" or other approved medications.[14] If those methods fail, an animal is culled (removed) and—if given antibiotics or other unapproved forms of treatment—no longer retains its organic status.

Whether or not the agricultural use of antibiotics has an effect on humans, the small amount of organic meat and poultry currently raised in the United States will have little impact on the overall picture of antibiotic resistance.[15] But increased consumer awareness of this potential problem (due in part to organics' popularity) may pressure the conventional industry to change its ways. By June 2003, consumer activism had persuaded the McDonald's corporation to advise its poultry suppliers to phase out the use of antibiotics. In addition, the National Cattlemen's Beef Association managed a campaign that has nearly eliminated the use of the antibiotic tetracycline in cattle feed, noting that all major feedlots have discontinued use of this drug.[16]

FOOD ADDITIVES

There once was a time when the idea of organic Cheetos or Oreos could not be imagined even in the nightmares of organicists. Those days are over. Consumers today may have little memory or awareness of the food additive/cancer scare in the 1970s, and they may just assume that organic foods do not contain preservatives, flavor enhancers, or colors.[17] The reality is that processed organic foods like macaroni and cheese, sandwich cookies, and lentil soup mix cannot sit on grocers' shelves without additives.

Among FDA-approved substances, most natural substances are allowed in organics, while most—*but not all*—synthetic additives are prohibited. Because modern consumers demand—and both organic and conventional producers supply—prepackaged, convenient food, the issue of additives is one of the quieter controversies regarding organic foods. Nevertheless, additives still have their detractors and remain a source of concern for some. Although cooking from scratch can be time-consuming, it remains the best way to guarantee additive-free food, whether organic or not.

HORMONES

Use of hormones in cows dates back to the 1930s, when researchers discovered that injecting them with a substance (later isolated and named BST) extracted from the pituitary glands of cows increased their milk production. Because the process of extraction was difficult and expensive, use of BST was limited until 1993 when the FDA allowed Monsanto to market its patented genetically engineered form (rBST or rBGH).

Today there are six hormones registered for use in conventional beef cattle and four hormones approved for use in dairy cows (see Aisles 4 and 5). *None are allowed in the production of hogs or chickens.* While their use in beef continues in the United States, a number of countries—most notably those in the European Union—have banned the importation of hormone-treated meat since 1989 (despite the fact the European Agriculture Commission has deemed their use safe).

Organic advocates claim that the "weight of evidence"

suggests that adding hormones to the food we eat disrupts the endocrine systems of fish, wildlife, and people. They rightly point out that any amount of added hormones—particularly if they are synthetic—places unknown burdens on the endocrine system and therefore should not be used.

GENETICALLY ENGINEERED ORGANISMS (GEOs)

Not since the nuclear 1950s has a technology held so much promise while simultaneously scaring the willies out of a lot of us. Supporters say that genetically engineered crops could play a vital role in feeding the world's hungry. Detractors point out that GEOs could permanently damage the food chain.

The idea that we can now take the genes from one species and place them into another raises alarm bells with environmental activists and consumers around the world. As with atomic and chemical advances, science and industry are forging ahead, even though questions about the possible consequences remain. This apparent lack of caution has led to one of the defining controversies in food production. Conventional agriculture in the United States and in other countries outside the European Union has accepted GEOs, despite criticism that they could create new allergens and viruses; increase pesticide use; contribute to antibiotic resistance; or alter nutritional content.

Genetic Engineering: Methods and Questions

GEOs are not all created the same way.[18] Several different methods have been tried, and we will discuss two of them here. The first, *microbial inoculation and fermentation,* is the more common; the second, *recombinant DNA,* is the more contentious.

Enzymes, yeasts, and cultures used in beer, bread, cheese, vinegar, soy sauce, yogurt, soda, and other foods are the result of microbial inoculation and fermentation. This method involves inserting snippets of DNA—the enzymes for making cheese, for instance—into bacteria (usually a harmless form of *E. coli*), then growing the DNA-infused bacterial solution in nutrient tanks. When enough of the altered bacteria are grown, the solution is pasteurized to kill off the bacteria, leaving behind the desired enzymes, yeasts, or cultures.[19]

Recombinant DNA—the so-called Frankenfood—grabs most of the headlines because it sounds more exotic and frightening. Taking genes from one species and putting them into another presents both physical and ethical challenges. Physically, the technique involves isolating "desirable trait" genes in one species and splicing them into the genetic code of another. Doing this requires a whole bundle of genes, each playing a role in getting the desired trait to "turn on" and off at the right time and place to effect a change.

Ethically, the question is whether we should respect nature's species "barriers" or recognize the fact that all living things are made up of the same building blocks. Whether genetic engineering is seen as "playing god" or as nothing more than a continuation of natural processes using the vehicle of the human mind, it is the *recombining* of genes

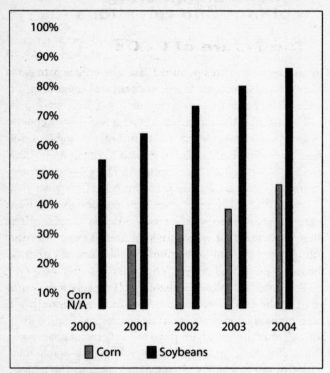

Growth of Genetically Engineered Crops in the U.S.

Source: Prospective Plantings: 2000-2004.
Agricultural Statistics Board, NASS, USDA

that critics claim creates totally new organisms. And eating anything new can be a risky endeavor, whether it's genetically engineered or not.

Despite the concerns of organic advocates—allergies, viruses, contamination of the food supply—"opponents of genetically modified food will not accept as evidence that the number of people who have eaten genetically modified food now number into the hundreds of millions without there being a single verified instance of even the slightest hint of harm to anybody."[20]

The Future of GEOs

Organic advocates point out that the only way to avoid GEOs is to buy organic food. Unfortunately, even organic foods may not be GEO free, because organic crops can be contaminated with pollen from nearby GEO crops. To combat the problem of genetic drift, the possibility of setting tolerance levels for GEO contamination in organic food is being discussed, although the NOP rule includes no such provisions right now.

As for GEO supporters, they have yet to make a clear case for consumer benefits, but even some critics who urge caution about biotechnology acknowledge potential future benefits. The issue remains a case of no definitive health risks and no obvious consumer benefits. However, the technology and the debate are both relatively young and promise to be one of the most volatile issues in the future of food production.

IRRADIATION

Conventional food processors, many scientists, and the FDA tout irradiation as an answer to the problem of food-borne pathogens. Although the prohibition of irradiation was not originally part of organic production standards, public outcry made it one of the "big three" issues. While organic advocates cite a number of problems associated with irradiation, public knowledge of the process and related health issues remains vague at best.

Currently, the food industry uses irradiation to:

- Kill insects, bacteria, and mold in spices, herbs, and vegetable seasonings
- Prevent potatoes from sprouting in storage
- Control beetles, moths, and weevils in grains
- Kill exotic pests found on imported fruit
- Kill the microorganisms responsible for food spoilage
- Kill the pathogenic microorganisms that make us sick

Conventional thinking claims that irradiation is safe, while organic advocates point out several problems. Like other industrial food-production technologies such as pesticides and GEOs, organic advocates see irradiation as a food-altering technological quick fix for systemic failures. In other words, the most often cited reason for using irradiation—dirty meat-processing facilities—constitutes the real problem (see Aisle 5).

While organic advocates have a point about the reasons for the use of irradiation, the low doses used on most foods have about as much effect on food as a sunny day has on us. But in higher doses the potential problems warrant attention. For example, irradiated potatoes are a pretty low risk, while frozen hamburger patties present a moderate risk.

NUTRITIONAL QUALITY

Ancient farmers knew from experience that manure made plants grow better, but they didn't understand why. Today soil science tells us that the elemental nutrients found in manure are essential for plant development. Three of these nutrients—nitrogen, phosphorus, and potassium—are considered most important,[21] but other minor nutrients and the organic matter in manure also play important roles in the complicated world of plant nutrition. Growing crops year after year on the same piece of land depletes the soil's nutrients, reducing a crop's yield and its nutritional content. This is a scientific fact, and there is no debate on this point.

The real question here is whether using synthetic chemical fertilizers reduces the nutrient content of food crops. In a literature review, Dr. Virginia Worthington concluded that "organic crops contained significantly more vitamin C, iron, magnesium, and phosphorus and significantly less nitrates than conventional crops."[22] But Dr. Ruth Kava of the American Council on Science and Health disagrees: "Dr. Worthington made a valiant effort to show that organic methods produce nutritionally superior produce, but the data simply are not strong enough to allow her legitimately to do so."[23]

Worthington's claims reflect the wishes of organic advocates to find one of organics' holy grails: some conclusive and irrefutable evidence that organic production methods produce food that is better for you. Thus far, some studies have shown slightly higher levels of vitamins and antioxidants in certain foods, such as organic ketchup, which has more of the antioxidant lycopene.

MYCOTOXINS

Unless you're a dairy farmer, a peanut farmer, or a health professional, you probably haven't even heard of these things. Mycotoxins are poisonous compounds produced by a variety of molds. For the most part, modern science ignored the mycotoxin problem until a hundred thousand turkeys suddenly died in southern England. Shortly thereafter, another two hundred thousand met the same fate in other countries. The culprit was found in the turkeys' dinner: ground peanut meal infected with aflatoxin from the mold *Aspergillus flavus*.

Since then health officials have taken mycotoxins very seriously because they are highly carcinogenic or outright poisonous to humans. Over fifteen different mold species can produce mycotoxins in food crops and livestock feed. Although the greatest threat from mycotoxins is found in food imported from developing countries where shoddy surveillance procedures cause concern, food production in the United States is not immune. American health officials take aflatoxin so seriously that the tolerance level in milk is only 0.5 parts per billion (ppb),[24] and government officials inspect other susceptible foodstuffs destined for human consumption.

Because organic production methods do not allow the use of most fungicides, critics raise the concern that organic crops may be more susceptible to molds. Unfortunately, only a few studies have been completed comparing the mold found on conventional versus organic crops. Some have found more toxins on organic food, while others have found less. The current consensus is that there is no more cause for concern in organic than in conventional food *at the present rate* of organic production.

Although the occurrence is statistically rare, peanut butter is probably the most significant source of mycotoxins, so the USDA's Peanut Marketing Agreement demands no visible mold and less than 15 ppb of aflatoxin on peanuts at the point of sale.[25] Because *Aspergillus flavus* can still grow after that point, several new testing methods and pesticides have been developed to limit the amount of aflatoxin found in the food supply.

PATHOGENS

Although you can take steps to avoid food poisoning, pathogens pose a more direct threat to your health than all the other issues discussed in this chapter combined. While organic production methods may significantly reduce the chances of encountering some pathogens, buying organic does not guarantee you pathogen-free food.

Pathogens are equal-opportunity infectors, but it appears that certain conventional food-production techniques—overcrowded livestock confinement operations, antibiotic abuse, and modern livestock feed—have encouraged disease-causing organisms to mutate into more harmful forms. Organic advocates claim that because organic food exists outside of this system, it is immune to its ills. This claim is not entirely accurate. One of the causes of harmful mutations—feeding ruminants high-protein grains such as corn—is not prohibited in organic standards. Food poisoning caused by microorganisms could potentially affect both organic and conventional products.

TO BUY OR NOT TO BUY

There are real concerns when it comes to the way our food is grown and processed, and it is easy to understand that the media attention given to organic food usually involves issues of health. Whether food safety regulations currently in place adequately protect us remains an open question. If you have children, your concerns heighten, and you often find yourself confused by all the conflicting media coverage. Do you reach for organic products every time, or only when your budget allows? For many parents, the question comes down to whether you spend your children's future college funds buying organic foods today. However you feel about science or the government's record of regulation, living is a continuous exercise in risk analysis, and when it comes to food, reducing risk may not hurt anything but your pocketbook. But if fear of modern food leads you to limit your intake of fresh fruits and vegetables, then you haven't done your body any favors.

If you have an unlimited food budget, buy organic. If, however, the higher prices give you pause, the guidance offered in the Aisle chapters should help you make more informed choices.

CHAPTER 4
Organic Foods and the Environment

HEALTH CONCERNS REPRESENT the public face of organics, but for most farmers, the story is in the soil, water, and air. Michael Pollan's assessment that "it has always been easier to make the environmental case for organic food than the health case"[1] speaks to the fact that organic standards—and particularly the standards practiced by small organic farmers—provide a blueprint for a more sustainable agricultural environment.

Any form of agriculture puts some strain on ecosystems. As the human population increases, so do the environmental problems related to food production. Conventional proponents seek solutions in large-scale efficiency, synthetic fertilizers, pesticides, and new technology. Organic advocates contend that these "solutions" are not sustainable and that industrial food production greatly exacerbates (or has created) the following problems:

- Degradation of land
  - Loss of soil fertility
  - Loss of soil life
  - Soil erosion
  - Soil salinity
  - Desertification (overgrazing)
- Degradation of water
  - Water contamination

- Degradation of air
  - Greenhouse gas emissions
- Lack of biodiversity
  - Loss of crop varieties
  - Loss of habitat
  - Genetically engineered crops

In this chapter, we look closely at the environmental impact of conventional food production and highlight ways in which organic practices differ. Since size is an important component of environmental impact, we make a further distinction between large-scale (industrial) organic, and small-farm (traditional) organic. In each of these broad areas, we offer an environmental report card for conventional agriculture, industrial organic, and traditional organic.

INFINITE POSSIBILITIES, LIMITED GARLIC

While planting garlic in premade holes, I (Luddene) ran short of cloves. Buddy, the free-range farm dog, was the only one around, so I offered him my assessment that I had a finite amount of garlic and an infinite amount of unfilled space. He didn't seem to care much, but the word *finite* reminded me of a conversation I had with my young son years before. He was concerned that all the new people being born would make the earth weigh too much and throw it out of orbit.

So we had the talk about conservation of matter.

As a way to explain that *all nutrients are finite and are simply recycled over and over,* I told him that elemental nitrogen (N_2) is essential to plant growth and makes up about 78 percent of the air we breathe. Unfortunately, most plants can't breathe N_2. The bean family is an exception and can take nitrogen out of thin air. Together with the symbiotic bacteria living close to their roots, they can convert N2 into usable plant-ready nitrogen.

This conversion takes place naturally in other ways. Soil microorganisms in conjunction with organic matter also do this trick—hence Howard's fascination with compost (and the whole foundation for organic farming). Since the late 1800s, human beings have figured out a way to do it with an industrial process (see Chapter 2). But no matter how it happens, there is only so much nitrogen, and farming wouldn't be possible without it.

To enrich soil, farmers can either buy NH3 in the form of chemical fertilizers (anhydrous ammonia, for example) or expend the labor to plant legumes (beans), plow in organic matter, or add manure. Although animal manure contains some nitrogen, it cannot match chemical fertilizer pound for pound. Here's how they compare:

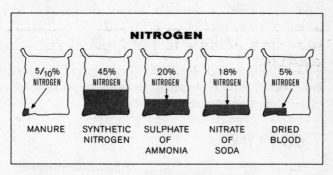

NITROGEN

| 5/10% NITROGEN | 45% NITROGEN | 20% NITROGEN | 18% NITROGEN | 5% NITROGEN |
| MANURE | SYNTHETIC NITROGEN | SULPHATE OF AMMONIA | NITRATE OF SODA | DRIED BLOOD |

The second component in the equation is protein—there's only so much of that, too. Protein has always been scarce and expensive. Today's expansive livestock industry wouldn't exist without a cheap source of protein: soybeans, corn, or rendered animal parts. The fact that nitrogen and protein are finite resources more difficult to obtain naturally is one reason that foods derived from animal proteins cost more.

DEGRADATION OF LAND

Soil Fertility

Unless you happen to be a soil scientist or a farmer, it's easy to fly over or drive through the vast swaths of America's heartland and take soil for granted. In the supermarket, we rarely contemplate that behind every food is a nutrient-rich soil. Not treating soil like dirt, by maintaining the land's productivity, is farming's most elemental challenge.

The many approaches for building soil fertility reflect the profound philosophical differences between organic and conventional thinking about the soil. Organic growers regard the soil as a living thing that requires nurturing. To them, merely adding chemical fertilizer short-circuits the natural soil-building process, pollutes ground and surface water, and is ultimately not sustainable. Soil, in this view, is more than the sum of chemical parts. Conventional proponents, by contrast, see the soil as made up of elements. For them, nitrogen is nitrogen, whether it comes from cow manure or a tank of anhydrous ammonia.

Soil Life

Closely related to soil fertility is the maintenance of a vibrant and diverse soil life. Billions of bacteria, fungi, protozoa, algae, nematodes, and earthworms live in topsoil. Their various actions have numerous benefits. Without these organisms, plants cannot effectively use nutrients.

Organic and conventional thinking differs somewhat on this issue. Although both sides acknowledge the importance of soil biodiversity, organic advocates claim that the heavy use of agricultural chemicals "kills the soil" and throws the intricate food web out of balance. For example, mycorrhizae help plants use nitrogen. When nitrogen fertilizer is injected into the soil, these fungi die, and plants become less efficient at using (fixing) nitrogen. Conventional proponents, however, contend that soil life rebounds quickly.

Soil Erosion

Caused either by wind or water, erosion is the loss of topsoil—where nutrients, microbes, and organic matter reside. Some soil erosion is a natural process that varies depending on landscape, vegetation, and weather.* In a healthy ecosystem, soil loss is minimal, but agriculture disrupts this natural state by exposing the soil to wind and rain.[2] Because fertile topsoil requires hundreds of thousands of years to form, erosion has been a serious problem for farmers since agriculture began. Over time significant soil losses diminish the land's productivity and cause a number of other problems such as excess dust in the atmosphere or silt in streams, rivers, and reservoirs.

Although soil loss is difficult to measure, the USDA's National Resource Conservation Service (NRCS)—the modern incarnation of the Soil Conservation Service—has been monitoring it since the late nineteenth century. The most recent long-term studies began in the 1980s, with data collected and analyzed every five years. The results are encouraging, showing a decrease in soil erosion since the study began.[3]

Improvements in erosion control in the United States have been the result of modern tilling techniques in conventional agriculture and better land-management strategies such as contour plowing. We point this out to note

---

* The states of Louisiana and Mississippi are the result of soil erosion beginning thousands of years ago.

that, while problems with industrial agriculture do exist, positive changes occur, because both conventional and organic farmers recognize that maintaining good soil is the foundation of any farm. All farmers have a vested interest in keeping their soil and so employ many of the same strategies; but there are some important differences between organic and conventional approaches to erosion control.

For organic growers, better soil and greater crop diversity make use of nature's own methods to prevent soil erosion. Conventional thinking sees the use of agricultural chemicals as a solution. By increasing yields on existing farmland, they say, conventional methods reduce the need to cultivate new, often less stable soil for food production. In addition, the use of herbicides also reduces the need to till weeds mechanically, cutting down on fuel consumption and greenhouse gas emissions.*

Soil Salinity

When the salt content in soil gets too high, plants cannot grow. This happens for a variety of reasons and is generally more problematic in arid or semiarid landscapes. The most direct agricultural cause of salinity is irrigation. As water evaporates, it leaves behind minerals. In time, more salt amasses than the crops can tolerate, making land useless for farming.

A prime example of soil salinity problems occurs in California's Central Valley, where temperatures are suitable for year-round growing but irrigation is necessary. Since both

---

* There is both an upside and downside to this point. Herbicides reduce the amount and frequency of tillage, keeping mechanical disruption of the soil at a minimum. Of course, given the inevitability of some erosion, the herbicides used may end up in ground and surface water.

conventional and organic methods rely on irrigation, the issue is not hotly debated, but traditional organic growers may question the need for growing crops in areas where agriculture is dependent on irrigation.

Desertification

When an arid or semiarid landscape can no longer support its natural vegetation, desertification occurs. Human causes include overgrazing cattle and other poor land-management practices. In the United States, this phenomenon largely results from our love of beef. Range cattle roam freely on the lands of the arid West, munching the vegetation to the point where the natural ecosystem can no longer maintain plant growth. Although the western range appears to be an immense hostile, sturdy, and useless terrain, it is in fact an extremely fragile landscape easily subject to erosion and vegetation loss. Millions of grazing cattle have destroyed much of the original condition of the area.

Although not directly an organic-versus-conventional issue, the practice of raising cattle on fragile terrain is part of the modus operandi of industrial agriculture. In the eyes of traditional organic advocates, it is another in a long line of unsustainable practices.

Report Card: Land

Problem	Cause	Conventional Agriculture	Industrial Organic	Traditional Organic
Soil Fertility	nutrient input	B (synthetic)	B (nonsynthetic)	C (nonsynthetic)
	rotation	C-	B	A
	green manure	D	B	A
Soil Life	agricultural chemicals	C-	B	A
Soil Erosion	cultivation	D (no-till: B)	D	D
	cover cropping	C	B	A
Soil Salinity	irrigation	C	C	B
Desertification	overgrazing	D	C	B

DEGRADATION OF WATER

Water Contamination

Agricultural byproducts—pesticides, fertilizers, and animal waste—seep into ground and surface water, threatening birds, fish, beneficial insects such as bees, and human beings.

Groundwater contamination results from chemicals moving down through the soil in a process known as leaching. The impact is especially problematic in agricultural regions during the growing season, but eventually it spreads to wider areas by poisoning the aquifers (underground lakes) that supply most of the country's municipal drinking water. The most pressing of concerns involves contamination by synthetic fertilizers and herbicides. The map on page 71

NITRATES & PESTICIDES: GROUNDWATER CONTAMINATION & MAJOR ASSOCIATED CROPS

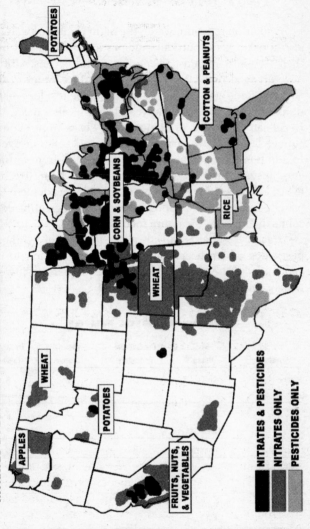

POTATOES

COTTON & PEANUTS

CORN & SOYBEANS

RICE

WHEAT

WHEAT

POTATOES

APPLES

FRUITS, NUTS, & VEGETABLES

NITRATES & PESTICIDES

NITRATES ONLY

PESTICIDES ONLY

shows areas of vulnerability to agriculture chemical contamination.

In addition to groundwater, the nation's surface water is also at risk. Excess nutrients and pesticides eventually find their way into streams, rivers, lakes, and oceans. Critics have charged that 90 percent of all surface water in the United States now contains some pesticide residues—and during certain times of the year, these levels exceed the EPA's safe levels for drinking water. Leaks from manure storage lagoons have polluted hundreds of miles of rivers. In addition, nitrogen and phosphorus runoff from fertilizers causes excess amounts of algal growth in streams, lakes, and coastal waters. These algal blooms deplete the water's oxygen supply, killing marine life and creating dead zones that disrupt the entire food chain.

Organic standards do not allow the use of synthetic pesticides or fertilizers, and therefore conversion to organic agriculture would address these problems if it were widely employed.

Report Card: Water

Problem	Cause	Conventional Agriculture	Industrial Organic	Traditional Organic
Groundwater Contamination	pesticides	C-	B	A
	synthetic fertilizers	D	A	A
	manure	B	C	C
Surface Water Contamination	pesticides	D	B	A
	synthetic fertilizers	D	A	A

Problem	Cause	Conventional Agriculture	Industrial Organic	Traditional Organic
	manure:			
	nitrates	D	C	C
	antibiotics	D	A	A
	hormones	D	A	A
	phosphorus	C	C-	D

DEGRADATION OF AIR

Greenhouse Gas Emissions

The prevailing winds of atmospheric science suggest that human contributions of the major greenhouse gases—carbon dioxide, methane, and nitrous oxide—are heating up the earth. Agriculture bears some responsibility for this problem in a number of different ways, but the most immediately recognizable contribution to greenhouse gases derives from the global industrial food system: moving products from food-producing regions to urban centers means the expenditure of fossil fuels.

While most consumers can understand the effects of transporting food, it's harder to see that the production of livestock and crops accounts for more than half of the emissions of greenhouse gases related to human activities.[4] Cows produce significant amounts of methane as a by-product of digestion, while nitrous oxide escapes from manure piles, waste lagoons, and fertilizers.[5]

Traditional organic practices may offer a remedy by encouraging local food systems, but *industrial organic* partakes of the same transportation system as conventional food. Buying local whenever possible is the only remedy for this problem.

Report Card: Air

Problem	Cause	Conventional Agriculture	Industrial Organic	Traditional Organic
Carbon Dioxide	farm equipment	D	D	D
	fertilizer manufacture	D	A	A
	transportation	D	D	B
	processing	D	D	B
Methane	livestock	D	D	B
	rice farming	C	C	A
Nitrous Oxide	fertilizers	C	A	A
	manure	F (feedlots)	C	B

LACK OF BIODIVERSITY

Loss of Crop Varieties

With the ever-increasing variety of food products in supermarkets, consumers may find it hard to understand that we are producing fewer varieties of food crops. Of the estimated eighty thousand edible plant species, we cultivate about 150. Industrial agriculture depends on a relatively small number of plants and animals bred from tens of thousands of wild and previously domesticated varieties. For example, the number of field crops—the staples of world agricultural production—has effectively been reduced to four: corn, wheat, rice, and soybeans. In addition, the gene pools of the big four crops have been consistently narrowed over the years through traditional breeding techniques.

While planting large acreages with a single crop defines

industrial agriculture and is responsible for the efficiency of production,[6] it is the primary reason for the loss of bio-diversity. To counter this trend, small local organic growers produce a wider array of fruits, vegetables, and grains and often specialize in heirloom varieties.

Loss of Habitat

While agriculture is not the only human endeavor responsible for the destruction of wildlife, many of the practices—deforestation, irrigation, monocropping—exact a toll on the natural environment. Conventional proponents take the view that some loss of habitat is the price of doing business, an "externality." Growing food carries inevitable costs. Organic advocates point to what they see as the real problem with industrial agriculture: it disregards all other concerns in favor of higher yields and higher profits. The ultimate goal of organics, they say, should be to develop sustainable systems with minimal impact on the environment.

Genetically Engineered Crops

Perhaps the most visible and contentious of all the environmental issues about agriculture is the introduction of genetically engineered food crops. Long-term effects on the environment are unknown, but organic advocates fear that GEOs will eventually contaminate all crops and cause mutations in weeds, insects, and microbes.

Proponents of GEOs seem unfazed by the grimmest scenarios conjured up by those who oppose their use. While they may acknowledge that some contamination is inevitable, they do not see it as a major problem. Organic advocates, on the other hand, see the transfer of genes across the species barrier as nothing less than a crime against nature, sacrilege—another in a long line of Faustian bargains made by science.

GEOs are not the only controversial area in the debate about bioethics. As far as their environmental effects go, we have only best guesses and risk analyses. For their part, proponents of GEOs seem exasperated by organics' adamant refusal to accept them, in part because of genetic engineering's *potential* to alleviate other known health and environmental problems. Organic advocates see a greedy crop science industry with a cavalier attitude about public and environmental health.

Report Card: Biodiversity

Problem	Cause	Conventional Agriculture	Industrial Organic	Traditional Organic
Flora	loss of seed varieties	F	C	A
	monoculture	F	C	B
	GEOs	F	A	A
	loss of wild plants	F	B	B
	potential gene transfer	C	A	A
Fauna	loss of habitat:			
	general farming	C-	C	B
	rice farming	B	B	B
	contamination of habitat	D	C	B

PLANET FOOD

Some of the practices favored by organic proponents play a role in easing pressures on the environment—the reduction of harmful chemicals and synthetic fertilizers being the most obvious examples. But it would be a stretch to say that organic methods offer clear solutions to all the environmental problems of post-industrial societies. Soil erosion is inherent to any type of agriculture, for example, but the mechanical weed control methods used in organic production may exacerbate the problem.

Despite charges to the contrary, the USDA has a long history of attempting to correct the ills triggered by agriculture. In 1894 it issued the first of many bulletins regarding soil erosion and its prevention. Moreover, it currently spends billions of dollars more each year to alleviate other agricultural problems such as well water contamination and manure spill clean-up.

In addition to measures already in place, organic agriculture can make a difference for the environment, but some of its solutions may also be problematic. While organics remain an important and laudable step toward a cleaner environment, considerable change would require a drastic increase in organic acreage, which in turn would mean a system bearing a strong resemblance to conventional agriculture. While traditional organic practices get high marks, industrial organic practices fare only somewhat better than those of conventional agriculture.

Final Report Card

	Conventional Agriculture	Industrial Organic	Traditional Organic
Grade Point Average	1.32	2.40	2.94
Final Grade	D+	C+	B

This is not to say that change cannot or will not come, but it will be incremental, built on decisions made every day by consumers. If concern for the environment is a high priority for you, look for local producers. Buying local is the greenest choice, and you can improve your options by making some small changes in your shopping habits.

CHAPTER 5
Organic Foods and Society

WHAT WE EAT goes beyond satisfying our physical needs. Food is essential to our cultural life and our sense of community. While industrial agriculture may provide abundant sustenance for much of the world's population, it often fails to address the values of social and economic justice held dear by many in the organic community. To them, the term *organic* reflects a set of beliefs and ideals—a philosophy that takes into account the health of society. Looked at in this light, organic agriculture rests on four fundamental principles. It must be:

- Nourishing: It produces healthy food and reduces potential toxins.
- Self-sustaining: It strives for ecological balance.
- Nurturing: It feeds rather than exploits.
- Democratizing: It seeks social and economic justice for farm owners, farm workers, and consumers.

When the USDA's National Organic Program developed its definition of *organic,* much of the philosophy was put out to pasture. To die-hard organic advocates, forsaking these principles left an empty seat at the world's dinner table. Put another way, some organic advocates view society's health as resting on this simple postulate: the type of food you purchase constitutes a vote for the system that created it. Buying organic, then, is a vote against conventional agriculture.

Just as early enthusiasts saw organic as a reaction to conventional farming, many modern advocates see it as an alternative to industrial culture. In the minds of some proponents, the underlying values of organic production provide an alternative to corporate control of the food supply. So, what exactly are those values?

To answer that question, we will examine some of the social problems with conventional food production and the remedies offered by an expanding organic sector. The ideas explored here are:

- Downsizing the American farm
- The price of efficiency
- From traditional to industrial organic
- Organics' place in the world

DOWNSIZING THE AMERICAN FARM

J. I. Rodale's original vision of small local farms had more to do with horticultural production than with agronomy.* After he coined the term *organic,* backyard plots of tomatoes and lettuce dominated the practice for the next forty years. With few exceptions—such as Walnut Acres—large organic farms did not exist because traditional organic methods are difficult (some would say impossible) to practice on a large scale. The smaller the farm, the more control the producer has over inputs and outcomes.

---

* *Horticultural production* refers to the growing of fruits and vegetables and is more closely akin to gardening than to what we think of as farming. *Agronomy* is the production of commodity crops such as wheat and corn.

Local and Seasonal Food

Contributing to this "small is beautiful" vision was the idea among early health food movements that locally produced food was superior to food trucked in from thousands of miles away. Not only is local food fresher and more nutritious, it requires far less fuel for transportation. Eliot Coleman, a working organic farmer, defines local food as follows: "Fresh fruits and vegetables, milk, eggs, and meat products can be called local if they are produced within fifty miles of their final sale. Seeds, nuts, beans, and grain can be considered local if they are grown within a three hundred mile radius of their final point of sale."[1] Given today's system of food production and distribution, this may seem like a radical definition, but it is a familiar notion to organic growers and farmers market patrons.

Inherent in the notion of small and local is the concept of eating seasonal food. Again, this concept has been lost to the average American consumer, who is now accustomed to the year-round availability of a variety of foods that were formerly unavailable for much of the year. Dyed-in-the-wool organic advocates would say that just because organic strawberries are available anytime of the year does not mean they should be. Buying organic produce from large nationwide markets may not fulfill the social concerns as organic advocates would have led us to believe. Helping small farmers and supporting a true economy are best accomplished when the source of your food is as close to home as possible. Eating seasonally helps local farmers all year long and with some effort can be accomplished in any region of the country (see sidebar on the next page).

UP FROM THE ROOT CELLAR

We have had a long-running discussion about the local and seasonal issue. It seems Dan likes bananas, coffee, and chocolate and can't imagine not eating tomatoes throughout the year. In his more idealistic moments, he insists that buying products from those regions does help to raise all boats in the global village—especially if one shops for Fair Trade goods.

Luddene hears this argument often, and she doesn't wholly disagree with it, but she also believes it doesn't excuse the fact that the United States could be doing a much better job growing and shopping locally and seasonally. For instance, carrots grow fine in Minnesota, as many local organic market gardeners will tell you. (They also grow well in many other areas of the country.) But most of the organic carrots purchased in Minnesota are grown in California by one megafarm and travel over a thousand miles to a state that can grow perfect organic carrots—if consumers simply demanded it be done.

And steps can be taken to ensure a year-round, local supply of many vegetables. John Fisher-Merritt, of the community-supported Food Farm, lives just outside decidedly untropical Duluth, Minnesota, where he supplies the local co-op and 250-member CSA with a wide variety of vegetables in a very cool and short growing season (110 days). In the winter, he uses a computer to assist Mother Nature in keeping his root cellar at just the right temperature to store potatoes, carrots, onions, squash, and other vegetables for year-round service to his customers. Not bad for the western shores of Lake Superior.

The point is that there are many alternative ways to provide for our food needs. We just need to look beyond doing business as usual. Every area of the United States could be more food self-sufficient. Farmers markets, community supported agriculture (CSAs), and local food co-ops are stepping up to the plate with local answers; we just need to meet them halfway.

THE PRICE OF EFFICIENCY

For many American urbanites, farming still evokes the image of a man steering a plow behind a team of mules. In reality, modern farmers have traded in the mules for $350,000 tractors, complete with air-conditioning, surround sound, and global positioning equipment. What did agriculture gain in this barter?

For one thing Americans now have the most efficient farming system the world has ever seen. In fact, agriculture is fast becoming the model of corporate efficiency as imagined by Archer Daniels Midland's "sponsor-mercials" on PBS: "What if we looked at the world as one giant farm field? In tomorrow's global food economy, every crop will grow where it grows best and ADM can link farmers to almost any market in the world. This offers a natural alternative to improve agricultural efficiency, make food more affordable, and feed a hungry world."

Two things ADM got right: efficiency does make food more affordable. America's citizens enjoy cheap food, and in many cases, food *is* being grown where it grows best. For example, the United States produces a fifth of the world's grain because America's heartland just happens to be well suited for growing wheat and corn. U.S. consumers benefit from this cornucopia because the system has achieved an unprecedented economy of scale. Until the 1980s, the world had never seen a hundred thousand chickens living together under one roof. Same goes for twenty-five thousand pigs. Bushels of the world's staple crops are measured in billions.

Proponents of industrial agriculture say food could be even cheaper and more abundant if the U.S. farmer had freer access to new seed and chemical technologies, unhampered by regulation. Restrictions involving animal welfare, waste disposal, farm worker safety, and livestock feed additives only hinder economic growth. Instead of regulation, conventional thinking says that market forces can be trusted to regulate the industry for the betterment of all.*

The Changing American Farm

U.S. farms	1900	2002	Change
U.S. population	75,994,266	291,000,000	+215,005,734
% of population farming	38%	1.8%	-43.2%
One farmer feeds	12 People	120 People	+108
Total U.S. acres in production	837,000,000	938,279,056	+101,279,056
Total acres certified organic	0	2,343,924	+2,343,924
Number of farms	6,800,000	2,128,982	-4,671,018
Farms over 1,000 acres	50,000 (<1%)	338,542 (>15%)	+288,542
Average acres	155	441	+296
Number of working draft animals	36,000,000	<10,000	-35,990,000
Number of tractors	1,000	4,600,000	+4,599,000
Bushels per acre: corn	28	143	+115

Organic advocates contend that the industry can achieve this so-called self-regulation and cheap food only by escalating farm size, eliminating independent farmers, and engaging politicians for more subsidies. They decry the loss of farmers and their farms as detrimental to our culture. Throughout the last half of the twentieth century, American farms have changed significantly. Yields increased,

---

* Those who extol the virtues of purely market-based solutions gloss over the idea that market solutions only truly work if consumers have "perfect information"—a very difficult notion, ironically made even more difficult in some ways by the "information age."

farms and equipment grew larger, and fewer farmers were needed (see chart on the previous page).

With their allegiance to small and local farming, traditional organic proponents insist that the loss of farms in the name of efficiency has led to the decay of an ethical, healthy food system. In other words, not just the displaced farmer but the whole population suffers because this "cheap" food ends up costing society in environmental clean-up, residue testing, health care, subsidies to farmers, and tax breaks to large agricorporations. When organicists speak of a "true economy," this is what they mean—and they raise a valid point.

Stock and Trade

Corporate involvement drives the economy of scale, providing the needed fuel for agriculture's growth: investment dollars. Today new farming ventures are usually not the dream of one farmer toiling by himself on the land. Rather, Wall Street investors now view scaled-up agriculture as a stock option. Organic advocates say this corporate structure of farms puts our food system at risk. But it is not true, as they claim, that many of our farms are now "corporate farms," implying that large multinational corporations outright own and manage a significant number of farms. Many family farms have incorporated for financial and inheritance reasons, but 96 percent of all farms are *still* family owned and operated.* And yes, many of these family farms are very large.

Instead, multinational agribusiness exerts control by determining acceptable crops, adequate harvests, and prices.[2] It has become the trend for industrial agriculture

---

* Some farms are multifamily farms that usually consist of grandfather, father, and son(s), or brothers working the farm.

to be both vertically and horizontally integrated in a concentrated system. This structure starts with the corporate-owned seeds, extends to processors, wholesalers, retailers (and their highly coveted shelf space), and ends with the packaging waste in corporate-owned landfills. Ownership of individual farms is not necessary when the system favors those who can integrate, consolidate, and play the "economy of scale" game.

Organic agriculture attempts to wriggle out of industrial agriculture's economic squeeze by creating higher profit margins for farmers. The higher premiums commanded by organic products allow producers to farm smaller acreages and keep farms in the family, enhance rural economies, and return control of the food system back to consumers. Many organic proponents also claim that because the organic movement exists outside of "agribiz," the system is changed for the better. Purchasing organic food is a vote for a smaller, saner system. Every farm converted to organic means fewer chemicals used, better conditions for farm labor, and a safer food supply.

FROM TRADITIONAL TO INDUSTRIAL ORGANIC

The question then becomes: Just how far outside the corporate system is the organic industry? By the late 1990s, demand for organic foods was exceeding supply, pressuring organic growers to adopt methods more closely aligned to the economies of scale achieved in conventional production. This meant increasing the number and size of organic farms. For example, one California purveyor of organic vegetables started in 1984 with less than three acres. By 1999, it had teamed up with the world's largest conventional lettuce grower, and the company now currently plants over 24,000 acres of organic lettuce.[3] At the local supermarket, the organic produce aisle mirrors its conventional counterpart, with nearly all the organic labels owned or controlled by the top five California organic producers.*

Corporate control of organic labels does not end in the produce aisle. By the late 1970s, many idealistic and dedicated individuals had developed a variety of processed organic foods like granola, pasta, bread, and soup. Most began manufacturing these foods simply because they wanted to eat them and found that they were nonexistent in the marketplace. Twenty years later some of these pioneers began cashing in by selling out to the same huge corporations that had evoked disdain only a decade or two earlier. Today the trend in all organic sectors has generally followed a familiar path—one that looks a lot like conventional food production.

What these large players brought to the table was more efficient manufacturing methods, a wider reach, and sophisticated marketing techniques that make some processed foods seem healthy because they contain organic ingredients—complete with an official seal. Large food conglomerates—often partly owned by even larger multinational corporations—own many of the most visible organic brands. The result: aging organic traditionalists find it inconceivable that the word *organic* now appears on packages of Tostitos.

---

* For a wonderful graphic presentation of this trend, see www.certified organic.bc.ca/rcbtoa/services/corporate-ownership.html.

The Problem with Industrial Organic

Growing the amount of organic food the market now demands requires more than just creating larger farms. Not all of the land that farmers have chosen to convert to organic is blessed with natural fertility. Good fertility can be developed and maintained by traditional organic methods, but it takes time—time to grow cover crops, time to adequately compost manures, time to till in organic matter.

But patience is not industry's forte. In the industrial organic world, production must increase *now,* requiring approved off-farm fertilizers. Inputs such as fish meal, chicken feathers, cottonseed meal, and bird guano supplement traditional organic soil-building techniques.[4] Even traditional composting techniques become problematic when, say, large organic vegetable farms haul manure from an organic dairy in another state. Although some of the off-farm nutrients are recycled agricultural waste products, others carry more onerous repercussions. The organic industry would prefer that the implications of these inputs remain buried. For example, does the world's fish population need further exploitation? What South Pacific island is being strip-mined for bird guano? What are the environmental implications of trucking thousands of tons of manure miles from its source?

Farm Worker Safety

Using off-farm nutrient inputs and trucking produce across the country are not the only organic practices being called into question by traditionalists. Planting, weeding, and harvesting all have one costly thing in common: hand labor. Someone must be found to do these backbreaking tasks. When it comes to field work, large-scale organic production practices follow the conventional model: using underpaid, seasonal migrant farm workers.

One meaningful difference for field workers on organic farms is reduced exposure to synthetic pesticides. On conventional farms, workers frequently handle chemicals, work in recently sprayed fields, or drink pesticide-contaminated water. Although acute poisonings in the United States rarely result in death, the EPA estimates that three hundred thousand farm workers suffer acute pesticide poisoning each year. Long-term (chronic) exposure at the farm level may result in higher incidences of some cancers and other health problems such as immune system dysfunction. Anecdotal reports from clinicians indicate that many cases of pesticide poisoning are unreported because patients do not seek treatment, or are misdiagnosed because the symptoms of pesticide poisoning can resemble those of viral infection.[5] In this respect, organic agriculture clearly offers a safer alternative.

On the downside, farming without synthetic chemicals involves considerable handwork. Nothing about hoeing, pruning, or harvesting is easy or injury free. Moreover, the pay rate for manual labor is still woefully below a living wage, which again brings up the question of social justice.

Animal Welfare

Another feature in the philosophy of organic agriculture concerns animal welfare. Public concern about the treatment of livestock continues to grow. In many cases, human health concerns—from BSE (mad cow disease) to *E. coli*—have driven consumer awareness about modern meat production. The growing popularity of organic meat has exposed more people to the conditions under which farm animals now exist. (See Aisle 5.)

Beyond Organic

Consequently, the question for many traditional organic thinkers is this: How can anything that is grown on huge farms, transported thousands of miles, intensely advertised, loaded with sugar (albeit organic sugar), and owned by some of the largest multinational corporations reflect the values they still hold dear? In their eyes, today's highly processed organic foods—when compared to their conventional counterparts—have more similarities than differences.

The whole trend highlights some glitches with the organic ideal. Success has had its price: the dilution of organic agriculture's mission to change the structure of the food system. Already new "beyond organic" labels are attempting to trump the NOP, and many traditional organic growers see this as the only way to keep their hopes alive.

One such attempt is Certified Naturally Grown (CNG). CNG calls itself a "grassroots alternative" to the NOP, a throwback to earlier days when certifying agencies formed committees of farmers to inspect one another. CNG insists that all farmer members adhere to the NOP's production methods, but it offers relief from the restrictive paper documentation and expenses that small-farm operations have trouble maintaining. Members of CNG are encouraged to market their products through farmers markets, roadside stands, local restaurants, CSAs (see page 136), and local grocery stores. Because the U.S. government now owns the word *organic,* use of that word on any product label not officially sanctioned by an accredited agency is in violation of the NOP rule. In addition, alternative labels (code words for organic) are "not permitted as *replacements* for the word organic" (emphasis added).[6]

ORGANICS' PLACE IN THE WORLD

The growth in organic farming and its products is a worldwide phenomenon. Canada, Australia, New Zealand, and the European Union all have acres of crops and livestock under organic production. Both Australia and Europe have a higher percentage of acreage devoted to organic practices than the United States. In fact, organic agriculture receives more government subsidies, marketing assistance, and research dollars in some smaller EU countries than in the entire United States.

Beyond the Northern Hemisphere and throughout the developing world, organic growers are organizing marketing cooperatives to promote their products in Europe and North America. The list of tropical organic commodities continues to expand. Twenty years ago many organic advocates attached some guilt to first-world consumption of imports such as cocoa, coffee, tea, and tropical fruits—pointing to the corporate control of indigenous people's lands, indiscriminate pesticide use, and the destruction of local food cultures. A remedy has emerged in Fair Trade, although it is not currently part of NOP regulations.

Feeding the World

Despite the small relief provided by Fair Trade, the problem of feeding the world remains a complex issue, and answers continue to elude us. Organic advocates place the blame squarely on multinational corporate control of the food supply. Conventional proponents claim that the only way to feed the current population of six billion people (as well as the projected nine or ten billion people by 2050) is to continue increasing yields on existing arable land using conventional methods and technology.

A Question of Yields

The Organic Farming Research Foundation reviewed yield studies from seven universities that totaled the results from 154 growing seasons.[7] It found that organic corn, soybeans, and wheat averaged 95 percent of conventional crops; other organic crops yield, on average, between 80 and 100 percent of conventional yields.

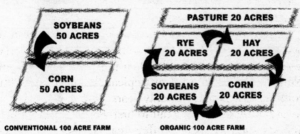

CONVENTIONAL VS. ORGANIC TOTAL FARM YIELDS (100 ACRES)

SOYBEANS 50 ACRES

CORN 50 ACRES

CONVENTIONAL 100 ACRE FARM

PASTURE 20 ACRES

RYE 20 ACRES

HAY 20 ACRES

SOYBEANS 20 ACRES

CORN 20 ACRES

ORGANIC 100 ACRE FARM

But "per acre bushel yield" is not the most important issue. The comparison should be made from total production of conventional farms to total production of organic farms. Why? Because in order to maintain yields, organic farms must create an extensive rotation plan that takes acres out of marketable food production. Oats, for example, may be harvested, but they are often plowed under to enrich the soil. Alfalfa is used for livestock.

In addition, many organic grain farms (corn, soybeans, wheat) also include livestock; most conventional commodity farms no longer do. The result? While the organic farmer's yield per acre compares to a conventional farm, there is significant overall reduction (see next page).

In the above example (a typical rotation for an organic

farm), it is easy to see that even without a reduction in yield per acre, the organic farm produces only twenty acres of soybeans or corn compared to fifty acres on the conventional farm.

Organic versus Conventional Yields[8]

Crop	Conventional			Organic		
	Acres	Bushels/Acre	Bushels Harvested	Acres	Bushels/Acre	Bushels Harvested
Corn	50	143	7,150	20	126	2,520
Oats	X	X	X	20	64	1,280
Alfalfa	X	X	X	20	5.4 tons	feed
Pasture	X	X	X	20	X	feed
Soybeans	50	44	2,200	20	37	740

When faced with this scenario, organic proponents in the United States insist this would all work out if Americans reduced their consumption of animal products, allowing for smaller farms with livestock operations. While this may be true, relying on Americans to change their food-consumption habits is problematic. The same is true for developing countries with rising per capita incomes. Where wealth increases, a desire for animal flesh seems to follow. Even if meat consumption did decline in the United States, the notion that small, diverse organic farms with livestock offer a viable solution is open to question.*

---

* Most areas of the country are fairly crop specific. Wheat needs less water than corn; thus it can grow on the arid high plains, and corn can't. Corn usually doesn't grow farther north than Fargo, North Dakota. And so on.

Here's how American agriculture would have to change to accommodate the organic model:

- It would need an additional 2,851,504 farmers.
- It would need an additional two million farmhouses and barns.
- It would devote 32 percent less land to corn, soybeans, and wheat and much more land to forage, and it would plow down crops for green manure.
- It would reduce U.S. corn and soybean harvests by possibly 70 percent.

Obviously, there are no easy answers. Proponents of conventional agriculture see further industrialization as the only way to fulfill the needs of an expanding human population. Included in this worldview is a continued reliance on synthetic fertilizers and pesticides, hybrid seeds, and genetic modification. Organic advocates claim these practices are unhealthy and unsustainable, and the way forward is, in part, a hearkening back to more traditional ways of farming.

THE VALUES ISSUE

For all the complications involved with assessing organics' potential influence on societal health, the question really comes down to this: What type of food system offers the most humane future? The two very different answers to this question reflect different values and ways of measuring success. Conventional proponents see success in numbers and efficiency, whereas organic advocates would like to see "quality of life" added to the equation.

Buying local whenever possible carries some obvious advantages. It more closely connects consumer and producer, physically, economically, and intellectually. Bringing food production closer to home strengthens community and communication. However, organic advocates would do well to continue paying close attention to conventional arguments about world hunger. Rejecting conventional innovations out of hand will only lead to further entrenchment and a breakdown in the necessary dialogue that must continue to take place for a more sustainable agricultural future.

PART II
Navigating the Aisles

WE SET OUT to determine if organic foods justify the added cost. But your food choices depend on your perceptions, your values, and your food budget. At the beginning of Part I, we asked you a few questions to help determine what kind of organic shopper you were. Now, with a wider knowledge of the issues involved in organic production, the following questions will help clarify and extend that earlier snapshot of your organic food-buying habits.

BUYER PROFILE

HEALTH

Circle all that apply.

In my opinion, organic farming methods ...

• Produce food without antibiotics, GEOs, hormones	1
• Produce food that is safer to eat	1
• Produce food with more nutrients	1
• Produce food that tastes better	1
• None of the above	0

I think organic foods are healthier, so I buy them because I am concerned about ...

• Pesticides, additives, hormones, etc.	1
• Obesity and overeating	0
• Pathogens found in conventional food	0
• Decreasing nutrients in our food supply	1
• None of the above	1

Since organic foods are healthier, I would buy organic …

• Candy bars	0
• Cookies	0
• Potato chips	0
• Packaged items	1
• Produce, meat, dairy	1

My biggest food-related health fear is …

• Hormone disruption	1
• Cancer	1
• Antibiotic resistance	1
• Food poisoning	1
• None of the above	0

Add up the circled numbers in each column,
then total them to get your Health Score

_____

ENVIRONMENT

Circle all that apply.

In my opinion, organic agriculture …

• Supports natural ecosystems and ecological harmony	1
• Will provide a better future food environment	1
• Builds a biologically diverse, healthy ecosystem	1

• Helps protect water resources	1
• None of the above	0

I think organic foods are better for the environment, so I buy them because of my concern about …

• Land degradation (erosion, overgrazing, etc.)	1
• Water degradation (contamination, depletion, etc.)	1
• Air degradation (greenhouse gas emissions, etc.)	1
• Lack of biodiversity (loss of habitat, GEOs, etc.)	1
• None of the above	0

I believe that organic farming methods can deliver on promises to …

• Feed the world in a sustainable way	1
• Reduce harmful greenhouse emissions	1
• Revitalize depleted soil nutrient levels	1
• Contribute to adequate and clean water	1
• None of the above	1

Add up the circled numbers in each column,
then total them to get your Environment Score   ____

SOCIETY

Circle all that apply.

In my opinion, organic food production provides a way to …

• Ensure farm worker safety	1
• Meet our needs but not at the expense of the future	1
• Help small farmers	1
• Support a local economy	1
• None of the above	0

I think foods farmed organically are socially responsible, so I buy them because organic farming methods are ...

• Nurturing—feed rather than exploit	1
• Self-sustaining—strive for ecological balance	1
• Nourishing—produce healthy food, reduce toxins	1
• Democratizing—seek social and economic justice	1
• None of the above	0

Keeping in mind the organics movement's philosophical underpinnings, I believe that ...

• Each dollar I spend on food is a "vote"	1
• I should eat locally and seasonally	1
• Industrial agriculture cannot be trusted	1
• Large organic farms address all social concerns	0
• None of the above	0

In the larger social context, I believe that organic ideals are best supported by purchasing food from ...

• Conventional supermarkets	1
• Natural food chains	1
• Food co-ops	1
• Farmers markets or CSAs	1
• It doesn't matter as long as it is organic	0

Add up the circled numbers in each column, then total them to get your Society Score ____

OTHER (WILD CARD)

Circle all that apply.

I will buy organic food products only if ...

• They are the best tasting	1
• They are the only ones available	1
• They are equal in cost	1
• None of the above	0

I think organic food is most closely related to ...

• Local food	1
• Gourmet food	1
• Ethnic food	1
• Specialty food	1
• None of the above	0

To me, organic foods seem ...

• Hip and trendy	1
• The best of the best	1
• Associated with the counterculture	1
• High priced, but okay occasionally	0

Add up the circled numbers in each column,
then total them to get your Wild Card Score   ____

Your score for each section is a ranking of the issues you most care about, and the type of shopper you are most likely to be (your Buyer Profile). For example, a high score in the Environment section makes you most like a Green Shopper. A high score in Health makes you most like a Healthy Shopper. And so on.

Category	Your Score	Symbol	Buyer Profile
Health			Healthy Shopper (Basic)
Environment			Green Shopper (Choice)
Society			Socially Conscious Shopper (Classic)
Wild Card			Your decisions may lie outside typical reasons for buying organic.

Now that you have determined your profile, the following chart, provided at the end of each Aisle, will direct you to the types of products that best reflect your ideas about how food should be grown and processed.

Buyer Profiles

 Healthy Shoppers: You see conventional foods as an unhealthy choice. You are concerned that the chemicals, antibiotics, hormones, etc., are too risky, and that by purchasing higher-priced organic foods, you are really buying peace of mind. For you, science and technology do not have all the answers and waiting until all the statistics are in is too long to stumble in the dark. Because health is your highest priority, you are open to even healthier options beyond organic.

 Green Shoppers: You live your beliefs. We have only one world, and you think your menu shouldn't be contributing to the end of it. You will buy organic if you perceive that it is the greenest choice. Other foods—local, seasonal, bulk—may also hold hope, even if they are not organic.

 Socially Conscious Shoppers: Your health and the planet's health are important, but so is the health of other people in the world. You believe the only way to improve society is by treating all of Earth's people in a just manner, and you seek out products that alleviate economic disparity, unhealthy conditions for food industry employees, and poor treatment of animals.

 Wild Card: For you, cooking is an art form. You are most concerned with the best-tasting, best-performing ingredients, and will buy organic only if it best fits your culinary needs. You do not have health concerns regarding conventional food, but you do dislike fast, convenience, and packaged foods.

AISLE SPECIALS

The Aisle chapters are designed to provide you with information about the different production practices behind the items you see on the shelves. Several other features will help guide you. Product Profiles (like the one below, for squash) contain a map showing the major areas of production and other relevant data about how each crop is grown:[1]

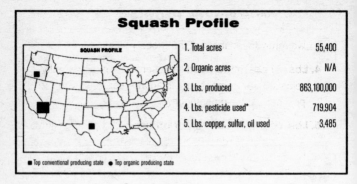

Squash Profile

1. Total acres	55,400
2. Organic acres	N/A
3. Lbs. produced	863,100,000
4. Lbs. pesticide used*	719,904
5. Lbs. copper, sulfur, oil used	3,485

■ Top conventional producing state ● Top organic producing state

Key:

- **The Production Map** indicates the largest areas of production. The large square indicates the place where the bulk of the U.S. conventional crop is grown, while the two smaller squares indicate the states with the second- and third-highest production. Organic production information—if available—will be marked with circles.

1. **Total acres** includes the total area devoted to growing both organic and conventional versions of a particular crop.

2. **Organic acres** represents the most recent figure—when available—regarding the number of acres under organic production.[2]

---

* Unfortunately, the most recently available data are from 1997, which makes our comparisons somewhat problematic. But pesticide use on major crops—despite what you may have heard—shows a downward trend since 1997. See www.ers.usda.gov/Briefing/AgChemicals/Questions/pmqa4.htm. This does not mean that the overall trend is reflected for *each* produce item. We encourage you to make your own comparisons when the latest data becomes available at the National Center for Food and Agricultural Policy's website: www.ncfap.org.

3. Lbs. produced attempts to put some perspective on the massive amount of food grown—a contextual perspective we rarely think about at the grocery store.

4. Lbs. of pesticide used represents the most recently released government data in an attempt to put the pesticide issue in perspective.

5. Lbs. of copper, sulfur, or oil used. Both conventional and organic production methods use copper, sulfur, and oil, a fact rarely mentioned in broadside attacks on pesticides.

6. Other relevant statistics for meat, dairy, and eggs, such as the frequency of hormone use in cattle.

In addition to the Product Profiles, each Aisle features Taste Checks; Best Bet charts, Organic versus Conventional brand comparisons for selected items; a summary of production differences; the Buyer Profile charts; and Brand Guides that include product logos and company contact information. The brand guides are included for your convenience, offering you a chance to browse through the aisles of gourmet shops, health food stores, local co-ops, national chains (like Whole Foods or Wild Oats), and—in some cases—conventional supermarkets. Some brands listed here can only be found in certain regions of the country, while others may be available nationwide or online. We have tried to include as many brands as possible, but the rapid growth of the industry and the regional nature of some branding (dairy, for instance) makes it difficult to include every organic brand available.

AISLE 1
The Produce Department

FOR MOST CONSUMERS, fruits and vegetables are the gateway organic product. Supermarkets usually stock organic produce before opening up shelf space for other items. And produce is the first item encountered in most grocery stores. In short, when consumers first think about organic, they think produce.

The National Agriculture Statistics Service (NASS) currently lists twenty-eight fruits and twenty-seven vegetables grown in the United States. All are grown organically, but some may not be readily available. Describing the growing methods for each one is beyond the scope of this book, so we've included a sample vegetable (tomatoes) and fruit (apples) to illustrate the growing, processing, and distribution methods that farmers depend on to bring their goods to the marketplace. We cover a few other produce items in the Product Profiles throughout the chapter. In addition, this aisle explores:

- Produce and the organic movement
- Pesticide residues
- Marketing produce
- Trends in organic produce production
- Vegetable production
- Fruit production
- Post-harvest treatment of produce
- Buying fruits and vegetables

PRODUCE AND THE ORGANIC MOVEMENT

Organic fruits and vegetables have been grown and marketed longer than any other organic product, and many industry pioneers cut their teeth on small market gardens in the 1970s. Earthbound Farms, the largest distributor of organic produce in the United States, began as a two-and-a-half acre raspberry patch in 1984. Today their lettuce is grown on 24,500 certified acres and is available in more than three-quarters of *all supermarkets* in the United States.[1]

Success stories like this one keep organic produce at the top of total sales for all organic foods, but fruits and vegetables no longer make up the *fastest-growing* segment of the market. Throughout the 1990s several other organic sectors—dairy, nondairy beverages, convenience foods, and snacks—surged ahead in popularity. By 2004, organic meat sales increased more than 77 percent.[2] Still, organic produce accounts for over $4 billion of the $10 billion organic industry, which is more than twice the revenue generated by the second-ranked nondairy beverage market.

Although it accounts for about 40 percent of all organic sales, produce does not take up the most cropland. With just 49,000 certified acres, organic fruits and veggies barely register in the overall agricultural picture, and they even pale in comparison to organic agronomy crops (corn and soybeans), which have staked out 291,000 certified acres located mostly in the midwestern states.[3]

PESTICIDE RESIDUES

Consumer surveys confirm that produce makes up the largest sector of the organic market because shoppers fear pesticides. Although other conventional crops receive many more total pounds of chemicals, the residues on produce get most of the attention. While pesticide residues in a box of macaroni and cheese are an abstraction, thoughts of residues are hard to dismiss when one is taking a bite out of a (poisoned?) apple.

To address this residual fear, several nonprofit organizations and consumer groups have singled out produce to demonstrate the dangers of pesticides, particularly the implications for children and infants. One such organization is the Environmental Working Group (EWG). It has compiled many years' worth of government pesticide information in order to rank produce.

While placing produce into "good to buy" and "bad to buy" lists may seem commendable, if it dissuades consumers from eating fresh fruits and vegetables, it has done the public a disservice. The research overwhelmingly points to consuming more produce, *even with residues,* as the best health move consumers can make—a fact included, if softly spoken, on the EWG website.

Organizations such as EWG deserve credit for bringing the pesticide issue to the public as long as they do not use fear as the primary motivating factor. When consumers hear about the millions of pounds of pesticides used, they are understandably shocked. For example, potato growers in 1997 used more than 100 million pounds of pesticides—a staggering figure.

Potato Profile

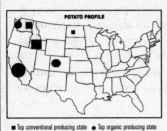

Total acres in potatoes, 2002	1,300,000
Organic acres, 2001	7,533
Lbs. of potatoes, 2002	46,321,400,000
Lbs. of pesticide used, 1997	101,154,067
Lbs. of copper and sulfur, 1997	2,889,692

■ Top conventional producing state ● Top organic producing state

But 100 million pounds of pesticides is only part of the story. Given the fact that the United States produces more than 46 *billion* pounds of potatoes each year, the pesticide use per pound seems less shocking. Moreover, critics of conventional farming seldom mention that oil and sulfur—two of the most widely applied pesticides—are approved for use on both conventional and organic produce.

When it comes to residues on food, a pesticide's purpose often determines the likelihood of residues. For the most part, produce ends up contaminated with insecticides or fungicides. Fruits are more likely to show up with residues than vegetables, although this is not always the case. Eighty-four percent of all potato samples contain chlorpropham—a herbicide actually sprayed on potatoes to keep them from sprouting while at the supermarket. This puts potatoes at the top of the residue list, because chlorpropham is designed to stay on the spud. (See the chart on the next page.)

Most Frequently Detected Pesticides on Produce

Rank	Crop	Pesticide	Type	Number of Samples	Samples with Residues	Percent of Samples with Residues
1	Potato	chlorpropham	herbicide (sprouting inhibitor)	121	62	51%
2	Apple	azinphos-methyl	insecticide	73	61	84%
3	Apple	captan	fungicide	174	60	34%
4	Apple	phosmet	insecticide	69	58	84%
5	Apple	diphenylamine	growth regulator	38	38	100%
6	Apple	thiabendazole	fungicide	37	37	100%
7	Peach	phosmet	insecticide	39	31	79%
8	Strawberry	captan	fungicide	41	24	59%
9	Apple	carbaryl	insecticide	22	22	100%
10	Peach	captan	fungicide	49	22	45%
11	Corn, grain	malathion	insecticide	39	20	51%
12	Wheat, grain	chlorpyrifos-methyl	insecticide	28	18	64%
13	Apple	4-(phenylamino) phenol	fungicide (metabolite)	17	17	100%
22	Potato	DDT	insecticide	127	12	9%
24	Celery	chlorothalanil	fungicide	83	11	13%
27	Green bean	acephate	insecticide	13	10	77%
28	Green bean	methamidophos	insecticide	13	10	77%

THE ORGANIC DIFFERENCE

Contrary to popular belief, organic produce farmers *do use* pesticides, but organic production regulations do not allow the use of synthetic chemicals. Despite the prohibition, organic fruits and vegetables are not guaranteed to be free of synthetic residues.

In August 2002, *Consumer Reports* magazine published an article detailing a study that appeared in the *Journal of Food Additives and Contaminants*. The article received a lot of fanfare in the national media. In a press release touting the research, the Consumers Union concluded that "seventy-three percent of conventionally grown produce contains at least one pesticide residue, while only twenty-three percent of organic produce does. Conventionally grown crops are six times as likely as organic ones to contain residues of more than one pesticide, the data show."[4]

On the surface, the news about organics and pesticides was good for consumers and producers alike, but the press release and article failed to mention that the study compared two quite different sets of numbers. While researchers looked at 48,807 conventional samples,* only 309 organic samples were used (less than 1 percent of total conventional samples).[5] Despite the good intentions and integrity of the researchers, this is only a first step toward conclusive science.

Looking Out for Produce

Although every state contributes to the nation's total supply, the vast majority of America's fresh vegetables are produced in California, Arizona, Texas, and Florida. California leads the pack by growing 48 percent of all domestic

---

* From the USDA's Pesticide Data Program, 1993–2002.

vegetables sold in the United States. Fruit production, too, tends to be limited to certain areas, but it remains more widely dispersed. For example, Washington, Michigan, and New York lead the apple-picking pack. While some of this concentration grows out of climatic necessity, the trend toward larger, more efficient produce-growing operations continues, and most of the organic fruit and vegetable brands distributed nationwide originate in roughly the same areas as conventional produce.

Imported Produce

Despite the abundance of produce, American farmers cannot supply the entire country's needs. Each year more produce is being imported from Mexico, Chile, China, and other nations. Cantaloupes and table grapes grown abroad now account for nearly half the U.S supply, and consumers naturally wonder if pesticide residues on imported produce pose a greater risk than produce grown domestically. Overall, the difference is not significant, but the question of inadequate testing remains open.

If residues are a concern to you, organics may provide an answer. Unfortunately, details about organic produce imports (as well as processed products like sweeteners) remain elusive. For example, China is the world's third largest exporter of conventional apples. On top of that, it has more than half a million certified organic acres, but there are no statistics available regarding the specific amount of organic apples imported from China—or any other country, for that matter. We can only speculate, but it's clear that demand for organic apple *products* outpaces U.S. production capacity. It's a good bet that some of the apple juice concentrate—a sort of universal organic sweetener found in processed goods—is coming from China.

Imported Organic Crop	Country of Origin
Dried apples	Moldova
Figs	Turkey
Pumpkin seeds	China
Dried pineapple	Mexico
Sun-dried tomatoes	Turkey
Almonds	Spain
Walnuts	Moldova
Amaranth	Peru
Buckwheat	China
Quinoa	Bolivia
Kidney beans	China
Lentils	Turkey
Safflower oil	Mexico
White vinegar	Italy

At issue for exacting consumers is whether they can trust the organic label on imported produce. Moreover, many ingredients in organic products are not identified as imported on the label. If it is difficult for U.S. producers to keep up with organic regulations, paperwork, and procedures, could the same thing happen in China or Moldova?

MARKETING PRODUCE

Years ago, before the United States excelled in mass-producing fruits and vegetables, produce farms ringed major metropolitan areas throughout the country. These small parcels of cropland were called "truck farms" because farmers would haul their produce into the city. For decades they sold directly to consumers, grocers, or street vendors and a farmer often knew who bought the fruits of his labor. Today that land supports the lawns and landscaping of suburbia, and produce is shipped in from greater distances. As demand for produce grew and production increased, individual farmers could not keep up with both the growing and the marketing of their crops. To help solve the problem, farmers organized marketing cooperatives in the 1920s.

For nearly seventy years, marketing co-ops, controlled by their farmer members, managed to provide good access to markets. Eventually, fruit terminals and produce brokers took over the majority of produce sales. Today most supermarket chains deal directly with packinghouses, which in turn have contracts with individual farmers. Contracts usually limit a farmer's freedom by dictating the variety of seed, the chemicals used, the planting date, and harvest deadlines. This leaves the farmer with little wiggle room, but also guarantees a buyer if the contract can be met.

While contract egg production has been in place since the 1950s, produce contracting has taken off only during the last decade. It would be naïve to assume that the large natural food chains ignore this system. Although some may make an effort to seek small local growers planting various varieties, the sheer size of these chains demands the efficiency of contracting through packinghouses.

Marketing Organic Produce

Before the 1990s organic producers dealt directly with natural food stores or the warehouses serving food co-ops. Selling an organic crop was usually a hit-or-miss proposition. Over the last decade, however, the large nationally known organic labels have managed to merge with the conventional system quite well. In fact, brands such as Earthbound Farms, Cal-Organic, and CF Fresh have morphed into large organic packinghouses, often related to multinational corporations.

While each started as a farm growing one or two specialty crops (in some cases, they still do), most now contract with both small and large organic farms that specialize in different crops. Contracting allows Earthbound Farms to market more than seventy-seven different fresh and pre-bagged fruit and vegetable products, while Cascadian Farms lists forty-five frozen and jarred produce products.

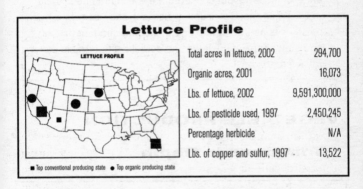

Lettuce Profile

LETTUCE PROFILE		
Total acres in lettuce, 2002		294,700
Organic acres, 2001		16,073
Lbs. of lettuce, 2002		9,591,300,000
Lbs. of pesticide used, 1997		2,450,245
Percentage herbicide		N/A
Lbs. of copper and sulfur, 1997		13,522

■ Top conventional producing state ● Top organic producing state

TRENDS IN ORGANIC PRODUCE PRODUCTION

During the 1970s small organic produce farms sprang up around the country, supplying food on a small scale to a very narrow band of consumers. Today most of the organic produce sold in supermarkets and natural food stores nationwide grows in the same places and under similar circumstances as conventional produce. In some cases, the very same conventional growers also market an organic line of products. Grimmway Farms, one of the world's largest conventional carrot growers with 34,000 acres, also produces the largest percentage of organic carrots (available under the Bunny-Luv and Sugar Snax labels).[6] Maintaining and inspecting the integrity of organic produce grown in these "split operations" constitutes a continuing challenge.

Taste Check: Carrots

We tasted machine-cut baby carrots, to compare organic and conventional. In the raw form we found no taste difference whatsoever, but cooked there was a dramatic difference. While most consumers use cut baby carrots as a relish or appetizer, others use them as a shortcut in soup and stew preparation. It was no contest—the organic carrots were the best.

VEGETABLE PRODUCTION

Tomatoes in Depth

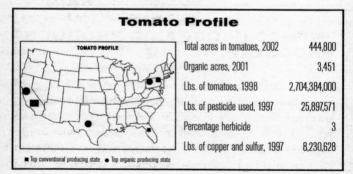

Tomato Profile

Total acres in tomatoes, 2002	444,800
Organic acres, 2001	3,451
Lbs. of tomatoes, 1998	2,704,384,000
Lbs. of pesticide used, 1997	25,897,571
Percentage herbicide	3
Lbs. of copper and sulfur, 1997	8,230,628

■ Top conventional producing state ● Top organic producing state

Most fresh tomatoes available to shoppers east of the Mississippi grow in Pennsylvania and Florida; California supplies them in the West. Tomatoes for canning, paste, and sauce also originate in California, but different growing methods apply: they are seeded instead of transplanted, the plants are not staked (no need to make sure they all look good), and mechanical harvesting takes the place of handpicking. Techniques for growing fresh tomatoes in Florida differ only in the types of chemical pest control used. Florida uses far less methyl bromide to control nematodes than does California. The following table details the distinction between organic and conventional production of tomatoes.

Tomato Production: Conventional versus Organic

Horticultural Need	Conventional	Organic
Planting Technique	Grown on poles through plastic, which is removed when crop is finished. Plastic is disposed in landfills. Wire is woven among poles to support plants. Plants are pruned and tied four to six times during the season. California farms also use bush varieties that require no staking.	Grown on poles or cages with various organic mulches; plastic is allowed if removed from field at season's end. Plastic is disposed in landfills. Large organic tomato farms weave wire among poles for support. Smaller farms use cages or other support systems.
Fertilizer	Of the 55 crops listed by the USDA, tomatoes are first in use of chemical potassium (K)—408 pounds per acre;	Organic consultants recommend 75–100 pounds of nitrogen per acre and "high" levels of

Tomato Production (Continued)

Horticultural Need	Conventional	Organic
Fertilizer	fourth in the use of phosphorus (P)—174 pounds per acre; and thirteenth in nitrogen (N) use—163 pounds per acre.* Application of fertilizer is incorporated in the soil before tomatoes are planted. Thereafter fertilizers are injected into the drip lines in a process know as fertigation.[7]	potassium and phosphorus. They suggest using 10–15 tons of manure per acre plus rock phosphate and mined potassium sulfate (K_2SO_4). All three are approved for use by the NOP.[8]
Weed Management	Chemical herbicides are used prior to planting. Subsequently, both herbicides and hand weeding are employed. Florida advisers list 14 different herbicides for fresh tomatoes.[9]	Organic farmers control weeds by rotating crops, using mulch, and hand weeding.
Insect Management	California tomato advisers suggest growers determine the "economic thresholds" before using insecticides. During 1997, 292,311 pounds of 22 different insecticides were used in California.[10]	Organic advisers suggest that crop rotations break the cycles of insects. In place of chemical insecticides, growers use insecticidal soap, predatory insects, pyrethrum, rotenone, *Bacillus thuringiensis,* neem, and ryania (all from natural sources).[11]

---

* Compare field corn at 56 pounds potassium, 57 pounds of phosphorus, and 129 pounds of nitrogen or soybeans at 68 pounds of potassium, 55 pounds of phosphorus, and 28 pounds of nitrogen.

Tomato Production (Continued)

Horticultural Need	Conventional	Organic
Disease Management	Fungi account for the major disease agents in tomatoes, and they can be serious. During 1997, 8.2 million pounds of fungicides were used in California, of which 92 percent were copper and sulfur.	NOP regulations allow copper and sulfur, even though continued use of copper can lead to toxic levels in the soil. Copper is also toxic to earthworms and some soil microbes.
Irrigation	All tomatoes grown in California are irrigated. Most now use a drip line buried in the row from 2 to 12 inches. Some furrow irrigation is still used. Most tomatoes in Florida are also irrigated with drip lines. Overhead sprinklers are discouraged because they contribute to disease.	Large organic tomato growers use the same irrigation methods as conventional growers. Smaller operations will use furrow irrigation or hand watering. Overhead sprinklers are discouraged because they contribute to disease.
Harvest	Harvest can last from 70 to 120 days in California. Fresh market tomatoes are all hand-picked, while processed tomatoes are mechanically harvested. Most tomatoes are harvested in the "breaker" stage, which means it is mostly green with some pink beginning to show.	Organic practices for processing tomatoes are the same as conventional. While large organic producers harvest fresh organic tomatoes in a similar manner, smaller growers selling in co-ops, farmers markets, or CSAs usually harvest tomatoes fully ripe.

Tomato Production (Continued)

Horticultural Need	Conventional	Organic
Post Harvest	Tomatoes are cooled to 55°F. to extend storage life to two weeks. Mature green tomatoes are then subject to the ethylene gas for 24 to 48 hours to induce coloring.	Organic practices are the same as conventional. Ethylene is allowed in organic production.

The production methods for each of the twenty-seven vegetables tracked by the USDA resemble tomatoes in terms of their general horticultural needs (column 1), although the details—chemicals used, climate, and processing methods—vary widely. All vegetables tend to consume more fertilizer, pesticides (per pounds produced), and labor than field crops.

BEST BETS: VEGETABLES

If you are looking for a way to cut down on organic produce costs, the Best Bet charts (which you will find in Aisles 1 through 7) provide a list of available vegetables and other relevant information. We have weighed nutritional value, price, and the potential for harm from currently registered pesticides. Our price sources were Whole Foods, Wild Oats, and Albertson's in January 2005.

Best Bets: Vegetables

Vegetable	Number of Current Pesticide Residues	Number of Environmental Contaminants	Availability of Organic		Price Comparison Per Pound January '05		Nutritional Value***
			National Brands*	Local**	Organic	Conventional	
✓Asparagus, frozen	8	2	L	W	$6.59	$5.44	M
✓Avocados	7	5	L	L	$1.69 ea.	$ .79 ea.	H
Beans, green	28	2	W	W	$2.49	$1.49	M
✓Beets	3	2	L	W	$1.49	$1.99	VH
Broccoli	13	2	W	W	$1.69	$1.00	H
Brussels Sprouts	15	1	N/A	L	N/A	$1.69	H
Cabbage	12	0	L	L	$ .99	$ .69	M
Carrots	10	3	W	W	$ .99	$ .75	H
✓Cauliflower	9	0	L	L	$1.99	$1.00	M
Celery	26	7	L	L	$1.99	$1.00	L
Collards	35	7	L	L	$1.99	N/A	VH
Cucumbers	16	8	W	W	$2.29	$1.00	L
✓Eggplant	9	0	L	L	$2.99	$1.99	L
✓Kale	3	0	W	W	$1.99	$1.99	VH
Lettuce	16	2	W	W	$6.05	$4.96	L
Mushrooms	10	0	N/A	L	N/A	$1.99	L
✓Onions	1	1	W	W	$ .89	$ .39	L
✓Peas, fresh	9	0	L	L	$3.59	N/A	M
Peppers, green	28	2	W	W	$2.99	$1.00	H
Potatoes	20	10	W	W	$ .89	$ .50	M

Vegetables (Continued)

Vegetable	Number of Current Pesticide Residues	Number of Environmental Contaminants	Availability of Organic		Price Comparison Per Pound January '05		Nutritional Value***
			National Brands*	Local**	Organic	Conventional	
Radishes	18	7	L	W	$1.49	$ .99	L
Spinach	23	9	W	W	$7.99	$4.00	H
Tomatoes	22	5	W	W	$2.99	$ .99	M
Turnips	10	4	L	L	$1.99	$ .99	L
Winter Squash	17	7	W	W	$1.29	$ .79	H
Zucchini	15	11	N/A	W	N/A	$1.79	M

✓=Best Bet for conventional

Source for Contaminants and Residues: FDA's Total Diet Study, 2002

* W = widely available; L = limited availability; H = hard to find; N/A = not available

** Seasonally available

*** L = low, M = moderate, H = high, VH = very high

If you are interested in looking at the lists of pesticides and other environmental contaminants found on food, see the FDA's Total Diet Study at www.cfsan.fda.gov/~comm/tds-toc.html. Further information about those pesticides can be found at http://extoxnet.orst.edu/ (Extoxnet) and www.panna.org/ (Pesticide Action Network North America).

FRUIT PRODUCTION

Most fruits are perennial crops like the apple tree, which can live for a hundred years (although commercial orchard trees are productive for only about twenty-five). This permanency means that growers must get off to a good start. Time and money prevent an orchardist from plowing down troubled trees every third season to eradicate a problem.

Fruit is an attractive food for both people and pests. While vegetables more easily adapt to organic production, fruit demands extra patience on the part of the grower. Small fruits—raspberries, grapes, and strawberries—often succeed quite well under organic production methods. But several persistent insects and numerous diseases like fire blight effect all tree fruits, and each fruit must also do battle with its own special nemesis such as peach mosaic or apple scab. In contrast to all other agricultural crops, fruit is plagued more by fungi than any other pest. In 1997, 84 percent of all pesticides applied to grapes were fungicides. By comparison, fungicides make up only 12 percent of the pesticides used on potatoes.

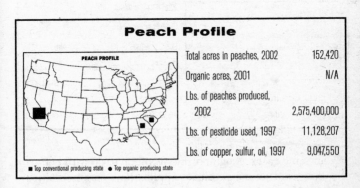

Peach Profile

Total acres in peaches, 2002	152,420
Organic acres, 2001	N/A
Lbs. of peaches produced, 2002	2,575,400,000
Lbs. of pesticide used, 1997	11,128,207
Lbs. of copper, sulfur, oil, 1997	9,047,550

■ Top conventional producing state   ● Top organic producing state

When it comes to organic fruit production, fertilizer needs can be met, weeds can be controlled, and commonly used fungicides like copper and sulfur are allowed—but battling bugs is another story. Insects such as the apple maggot and plum curculio may be particularly trying since effective organic solutions are few. Whereas conventional growers use Lorsban or Guthion to control these pests, there are no organic equivalents. The best that can be done against the apple maggot is to hang sticky red balls in trees to trap the adult flies before they lay eggs.

Before 1960 wormy apples were common, but today neither government regulators nor consumers tolerate such unpleasantries. Many shoppers have come to believe that picture-perfect fruit is normal. On a large scale, flawless, uniform fruits and vegetables exist because of intense management strategies that include pesticides. Gorgeous organic fruit is no different, and growers must constantly monitor their crops and take actions with NOP-approved inputs. Bad-looking organic fruit becomes juice, jam, or jelly.

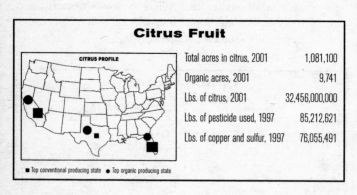

Citrus Fruit

CITRUS PROFILE

Total acres in citrus, 2001	1,081,100
Organic acres, 2001	9,741
Lbs. of citrus, 2001	32,456,000,000
Lbs. of pesticide used, 1997	85,212,621
Lbs. of copper and sulfur, 1997	76,055,491

■ Top conventional producing state ● Top organic producing state

In some cases, geography has as much to do with better-looking fruit as the pesticide applications common since the 1950s. The arid West simply has less pest pressure than eastern North America, and some of the most destructive insects do not thrive west of the Mississippi River. West Coast fruit growers, for example, have never had to compete with a plum curculio. (If you've never seen one, picture the Muppets' Gonzo.)

To alleviate damage from fungus, sulfur and copper have been used for hundreds of years and remain indispensable for conventional growers as well. For the most part, the relatively benign sulfur and copper ease persistent chemical pressure on the environment. However, these two organically approved and widely used substances elicit some criticism.

Andrew Kimbrell, writing in the 2002 book *Fatal Harvest,* expresses concern about farm worker health and safety while using sulfur. Many of the illnesses contracted by workers "involve skin and eye traumas from the use of 26 million pounds of sulfur dust, which is applied several times a year to nearly the entire acreage of California wine grapes. This sulfur dust has also contributed to widespread violation of the Clean Air Act limits." With nearly fifteen thousand certified organic acres now growing grapes, organic growers' sulfur use must also concern Kimbrell.[12]

Apple Production in Depth

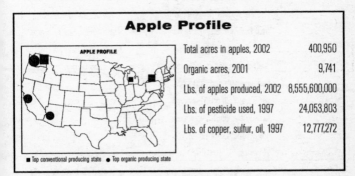

Apple Profile

APPLE PROFILE

Total acres in apples, 2002	400,950
Organic acres, 2001	9,741
Lbs. of apples produced, 2002	8,555,600,000
Lbs. of pesticide used, 1997	24,053,803
Lbs. of copper, sulfur, oil, 1997	12,777,272

■ Top conventional producing state ● Top organic producing state

During the 1970s any consumer standing in the produce section would have thought that the Red Delicious made up the entire pantheon of apples. In reality, 7,500 apple varieties grow worldwide (2,500 in the United States), but only about one hundred are produced commercially. Large organic orchards in Washington stick to the same popular varieties that conventional growers do. Small organic farms, however, experiment with hundreds of heirloom varieties.

Of the many heirloom varieties, most have dropped out of favor because they are low yielding, less pest resistant, comparatively small, or don't travel well. Commercial hybrids, however, often lack the flavor found in these exceptional old-timers. With good management practices, organic growers have capitalized on heirlooms. Look for them in specialty stores, farmers markets, and CSAs.

Apple Production: Conventional versus Organic

Method	Conventional	Organic
Planting Technique	Old orchards planted 100 standard trees per acre. These trees took up to 15 years to bear but were productive for up to 50 years. Today growers plant dwarfs and semidwarfs at between 500 and 800 trees per acre (called HDP or high density planting). These trees are productive for about 25 years.	Organic growers also plant dwarf and semidwarf trees. Large organic orchards in Washington state also grow the popular varieties that conventional growers do.
Fertilizer	Fruit, particularly tree fruit, are not heavy feeders. Overapplication of nitrogen	A significant amount of the fertility needs of fruit crops can be met through cover

Apple Production (Continued)

Method	Conventional	Organic
	causes serious fruit quality degradation, so it is rare. Most growers apply no more than 80 pounds of actual N per season to the soil no later than June 30.[13]	crop management and organic mulches.[14]
Weed Management	Weeds are not a significant problem in orchards. Many growers rely on clean cultivation to eliminate weeds. Only 7 percent of all pesticides used in conventional apple orchards are herbicides.	Orchard growers see weeds as somewhat valuable. They control erosion, provide a habitat for beneficial wildlife, and encourage pollinating bees. Excessive weeds may be mowed and trees may be mulched out to their drip line.
Insect Management	Of all the pests facing apple production, insects are the most devastating, both to the grower and to the environment. Fifty-eight percent of all pesticides applied to apples are insecticides, including chlorpyrifos, phosmet, and parathion.	Many insects that plague apples—scale, mealybugs, aphids—can be controlled with oil. Indeed, 78 percent of all insecticides used on apples—conventional and organic—is oil.
Disease Management	The most devastating disease any grower can face is fire blight. In less than a month it can wipe out a small orchard. Conventional farmers use antibiotics such as tetracycline	Organic growers are experimenting with spraying trees with harmless bacteria that outcompete fire blight. It's about 65 percent effective. Tetracycline is also

Apple Production (Continued)

Method	Conventional	Organic
Disease Management	to control it. Fungi represent a major portion of the diseases affecting apples. Thirty-five percent of all pesticides used on apples are fungicides.	approved for organic production. Organic orchardists rely on sulfur and copper as an effective fungicide. So do conventional growers— 27 percent of all fungicides used are copper and sulfur.
Other Pesticides	Some of the chemicals listed as pesticides used on apples really aren't pesticides. They are *growth regulators*. Like doggie treats, growth regulators get apples to do tricks. They can make apples stay on the tree or fall off the tree. They can make all the apples turn red at the same time. They even can make the little knobs on the bottom of a Red Delicious apple more prominent. This makes the real thing look more like its cartoon logo. The infamous alar was a growth regulator; it tricked the tree to induce blossom-bud formation. The most widely used growth regulator is ethephon.	The growth regulators gibberellic acid, indole acetic acid (IAA), and cytokinins are allowed for organic production. Twenty-two percent of all growth regulators used on apples are approved for organic production.

Apple Production (Continued)

Method	Conventional	Organic
Irrigation	Sixty-seven percent of all apples in the United States are grown in the West using irrigation.	Organic orchards in the West also use irrigation.
Harvest	All apples are hand-harvested, mostly by migrant farm labor. Washington state employs an estimated 44,000 workers to harvest apples; they reported earning an average $6.50 an hour.	Organic apples are harvested in the same fashion as conventional apples.
Post Harvest	All commercial apples are harvested when they are physiologically mature but not ripe. The apples are rapidly cooled immediately following picking and then are placed in controlled storage, where they can sit for up to nine months.	NOP rules do not prohibit the use of controlled atmosphere storage.

As with vegetables, the horticultural needs for fruit production apply across the board, but the details for each individual fruit differ substantially. Tree fruits, for example, are much different from berries when it comes to chemicals used; nutrient needs; harvesting methods; and post-harvest processing.

Best Bets: Fruit

Vegetable	Number of Current Pesticide Residues	Number of Environmental Contaminants	Availability of Organic		Price Comparison Per Pound January '05		Nutritional Value***
			National Brands*	Local**	Organic	Conventional	
Apples	34	5	W	W	$1.79	$1.00	M
✓Bananas	5	4	W	None	$ .99	$ .49	M
Cantaloupes	18	4	N/A	W	N/A	$2.00	M
Cherries	30	3	N/A	L	N/A	N/A	H
Grapes	25	3	N/A	L	N/A	$2.49	M
✓Grapefruit	7	0	W	L	$1.99	$1.29	M
Oranges	16	4	W	L	$ .99	$ .49	H
Peaches	25	5	N/A	L	N/A	$1.99	M
Pears	24	3	L	L	$1.99	$1.69	M
✓Pineapples	5	1	L	L	N/A	$2.99	M
Plums	21	1	L	L	N/A	$1.99	M
Raisins	21	6	W	L	$3.49	$2.19	M
Strawberries	33	7	N/A	W	N/A	N/A	H
Other Berries		—	N/A	L	$10.64	N/A	VH
Watermelons	11	2	L	W	N/A	N/A	L

✓ = Best Bet for conventional

Source for contaminants and residues: FDA's Total Diet Study, 2002

* W = widely available; L = limited availability; H = hard to find; N/A = not available

** Seasonally available

*** L = low, M = moderate, H = high, VH = very high

POST-HARVEST TREATMENT OF PRODUCE

Synthetic fertilizers and pesticides make up only part of the chemical assaults perpetrated on fruits and vegetables. Commercial agriculture—both organic and conventional—employs dozens of substances to ease the handling and maintain the qualities of fresh produce. Post-harvest procedures serve two main functions: to reduce food-borne pathogens and to prolong shelf life. To accomplish these goals, packers use some basic production techniques: cooling, washing, waxing, packing, and storing. Some produce varieties require all five, while others need only cooling and packing.

Cooling and Chlorinated Wash Water

By far, water, or "hydro-cooling," is the most common method of cooling produce. Although it cannot be used for all varieties, even small organic growers have access to water. This method—with the addition of other chemicals—also sanitizes the product. Packers use washing troughs called flumes that contain a disinfectant in the water to eliminate organisms that could degrade the produce or cause food-borne illness in consumers.*

Chlorine reigns as the most prevalent chemical in

---

* Pathogens causing food-borne illness may come from manure used in production or from equipment that was exposed to manure. But the most frequent source of pathogens in produce is field workers themselves. Although washing stations are now required in California production areas, it is nevertheless difficult under field conditions to wash hands on a frequent basis. It is easier for large operations to kill the bacteria on the produce than it is to eliminate it at its source.

flume water, and conventional produce bathes in as much as 150 ppm of chlorine during the early stages of the wash. NOP rules limit the amount of chlorine on organic vegetables at the end of the flume wash to 4 ppm. But recent outbreaks of salmonella, *E. coli,* and listeria have prompted some certifying agencies to allow up to 10 ppm.

While it is difficult to contaminate the inside of an uncut head of lettuce, processing vegetables into salad mixes now exposes all parts to bacteria. Limiting the amount of chlorine in wash water poses a potential problem for organic producers. On the other hand, bagged organic salad mixes (de-oxygenated and packed with nitrogen) may help cut down on the reintroduction of pathogens and preserve organic integrity. There is no evidence linking the use of nitrogen to human health problems, although salad mixes in bags can be up to ten days older than unbagged bulk mixes.

Chlorine ppm limits become an even more significant issue for alfalfa sprouts. Alfalfa can harbor *E. coli* within the seed itself, so the USDA and FDA have ruled that all alfalfa sprouts must be treated in water containing 20,000 ppm of chlorine. While that amount of chlorine eradicates pathogens, it far exceeds the NOP restriction on its use. Technically, organic alfalfa sprouts cannot exist. Despite the additional chlorine, contamination continues. In the summer of 2004, nine different companies recalled thousands of pounds of contaminated sprouts.

Chemical Soup

The term *flotation aid* brings to mind seat cushions in airplanes. In the produce industry flotation aids are chemicals added to vats of water (dump tanks) that force the fruits or vegetables upward and allow equipment to skim them off the top of the tank. Conventional producers use four chemicals: calcium ligninsulfonate, sodium sulfate, sodium silicate, and sodium carbonate. Two of these— sodium silicate and sodium carbonate—get the nod for organic production.

Conventional packinghouses also add other ingredients to dump tanks. Thiabendazole, captan, imazalil, shellac, and sucrose ester protect fruit between harvest time and consumption. Following the dump tank wash, producers apply a wax (usually carnauba or a petroleum-derived shellac) to keep the fungicide on the skin and prevent the fruit from drying out. Organic regulations allow carnauba, wood rosin, and beeswax but not the petroleum-derived chemicals.

Gift Wrapped

In addition to wax coatings, produce often gets wrapped in chemically treated paper. In the past, oiled or waxed paper controlled water evaporation from fruit. Today paper treated with oil, ethoxyquin, diphenylamine, copper, or a combination of the four protect produce in transit. Ethoxyquin can contain small amounts of p-phenetidine, arsenic, or lead, but most of the negative media regarding ethoxyquin refers to its use in pet food. Little has been said about its use in produce wrappers. The NOP rule allows copper but does not stipulate how it can or cannot be used in produce wrappers.

It's a Gas, Gas, Gas

Often used in grapes and berries, fumigation with sulfur dioxide in cool, sealed rooms destroys fungal spores on the surface of fruit. Some conventional produce is further subjected to ripening agents, such as ethylene gas, or the new mouthful: lysophophatidylethanolamine. Because some fruits—apples, pears, bananas, and tomatoes—are picked mature but not ripe, they can be kept longer.* Before delivery to supermarkets, ethylene gas initiates the color change associated with ripe fruits and is allowed in organics for post-harvest ripening of *tropical* fruit.

Apples Are Forever

One modern adage says that refrigerators are for storing food until it looks so bad we don't feel guilty about throwing it out. Every refrigerator has, way in the back, jars of unknown food items that have been there since the fridge was installed. Few of us, however, would keep apples in the refrigerator for nine months. Yet that's how long many apples remain in cold storage before their debut on supermarket shelves. It's called "controlled atmosphere" storage, and it's why we have Red Delicious apples in June.

To store apples, growers pack them in boxes, load them onto pallets, and keep them in refrigerators the size of football fields. Then all the air is sucked out, carbon dioxide and oxygen are pumped in, the temperature is set at 33°F, and the doors are sealed shut. Growers store apples because if all the apples came to market at once, the price would fall, and apples would not be available year-round—although imports from New Zealand and other countries have reduced the frequency of this practice.

---

* The life of fruit falls into four stages: pre-maturation, maturation, ripening, and senescence. Ripening begins to happen once a fruit has reached maturity. Enzymes in the fruit cause it to "breathe out" ethylene gas, which in turn effects changes in color and turns starches into sugars. Putting unripe fruit in a paper bag concentrates the level of ethylene and hastens ripening.

BUYING FRUITS AND VEGETABLES

We take for granted large displays of beautiful conventional produce year-round. Increasingly, this is also true of organic fruits and vegetables. From the consumer's standpoint, the produce aisle can be seen as a triumph of the global food system, but it does call into question some of the claims made by organic advocates. *If you are troubled by the health effects of pesticide residues or to farm workers, organic produce—regardless of where it is grown or how it is distributed—offers some peace of mind.* But if you are buying organic produce for other admirable reasons—"helping small farmers," "supporting a true economy," or "protecting farm worker health"—alternatives such as CSAs or farmers markets may more directly provide these benefits.

Your Local Co-op, Farmers Market, or CSA

One segment of the industry—local cooperatives—resists some of the trappings of industrial organic. Most co-op produce managers work with local farmers, and many food co-op bylaws and policies prescribe local buying. Still, organic vegetables available in the winter come from big-label packinghouses.

Another venue for buying fresh local produce is farmers markets. Even though certified organic products may not always be available—in one recent survey, *of the nineteen thousand farmers selling at U.S. markets, 47 percent offered organics*—farmers markets offer the opportunity to connect directly with local growers. Which brings up a thought worth contemplating: quality food grown by people who care may not always carry the official seal. Often the expense involved in becoming certified prevents small farmers from doing so, but this does not mean that their practices are not every bit (if not more so) as environmentally sound as large-scale organic operations.

During the last decade, more than 3,100 farmers markets have emerged in metropolitan areas throughout the country. Permanent markets usually operate Fridays, Saturdays, and Sundays during the growing season from May to October, while some markets in larger urban areas operate seven days a week and extend the season through December. In addition, neighborhood markets sprout up with portable canopies on Saturday mornings. Farmers markets offer an excellent alternative for consumers looking for tasty produce *and* a way to support small farmers.

For shoppers who wish to fully embrace the organic philosophy, community supported agriculture (CSA) offers exciting possibilities.* The idea behind CSAs is simple: members join by paying the grower up front for food produced that season. Members agree to take on the same risks and rewards as farmers. If a drought strikes midway during the season, members get less. On the other hand, a bumper crop might find members handing out fresh farm products to relatives and friends. Normally, CSAs supply a box of produce once a week for four to six months, depending on the length of the growing season in the area. In the warmer climates, CSAs operate all year long.

Some CSA memberships offer a number of different plans and pricing packages that usually run between two and five hundred dollars per season. Pricier plans including eggs or meat can usually be paid on installment. Work shares allow members to reduce costs and spend a day or two in the country experiencing firsthand how their food is

---

* The Alternative Farming Systems Information Center (of the USDA), at www.nal.usda.gov/afsic/csa/, is a great online resource.

grown (often cited by participants as one of the best features of joining a CSA).

Whether consumers choose a full share, sign up for a workday, or buy a onetime box, they experience a variety of fresh food while supporting a local grower. In supermarkets, consumers tend to buy familiar produce, but CSA members often receive lesser-known items such as kale, tomatillos, or radicchio. Most growers also include recipes, cooking tips, and other information about new vegetables.

Aside from their consumer benefits, CSAs also build strong regional food systems, keep dollars in the local community, establish a relationship between consumers and farmers, and further the task of changing the U.S. farming system.

Produce Production Comparison: Conventional versus Organic

	Conventional	Industrial Organic	Traditional Organic
Fertilizer	Vegetables: highest use of synthetic fertilizer of all crops	Vegetables: high use of purchased off-farm nutrients; some crop rotation; some green manuring	Vegetables: crop rotation, cover cropping, green manure, and compost
	Fruits: low use of fertilizers	Fruits: low use of fertilizers	Fruits: low use of fertilizers
Pesticide Use	Vegetables: low use of herbicides	Vegetables: no use of herbicides; mechanical cultivation and hand weeding	Vegetables: no use of herbicides, mostly hand weeding; more extensive reliance on mulches, rotations, and cover cropping

Produce Production Comparison
(Continued)

	Conventional	Industrial Organic	Traditional Organic
Pesticide Use	Fruits: high use of oil and synthetic insecticides; high use of synthetic fungicides and copper/sulfur	Fruits: high use of oil-based insecticides; high use of copper and sulfur, especially on organic grapes	Fruits: some use of oil-based insecticides; some use of the fungicides copper and sulfur
Pesticide Residues	Present in amounts deemed small enough not to cause harm	Found in about 25% of organic produce	Little testing has been done on small organic growers' produce
Marketing	Extensive use of contract growing, marketing pools, and grower co-ops; many brokers and terminals; considerable amount of produce production now controlled by retail grocery concerns	Some use of contract growing, marketing pools, and grower cooperatives; some brokers and terminals; a growing amount of organic produce now controlled by natural food grocery concerns	Local sales only, through CSAs, at farmers markets, direct at farm gate, or at food co-ops

Produce Production Comparison
(Continued)

	Conventional	Industrial Organic	Traditional Organic
Post-Harvest Handling	Widespread use of antispoilage chemicals; extensive use of disinfectants in wash water; packing materials frequently permeated with chemicals; produce frequently waxed; long-term controlled storage employed	Some use of copper and sulfur to retard post-harvest fungus; use of small amounts of disinfectants in wash water; packing materials not permeated with chemicals; natural waxes approved for organics; long-term controlled storage approved	Most produce harvested in the morning and is in consumers' homes by nightfall; small operations have neither the needs nor the capital for elaborate post-harvest processing

CONSUMER'S GUIDE

Aisle 1: The Produce Department

- Look for the USDA organic seal on all fruits and vegetables.
- Shop exclusively in organically certified markets or in markets displaying the GORP seal.

- Seek out local farmers markets.
- Buy local, unpackaged fruits and vegetables.

- Seek out and join a CSA or food co-op.
- Look for bananas and other tropical fruit with Fair Trade labels.
- Go to www.nal.usda.gov/afsic/csa/ for information about CSAs.

- Seek out tasty heirloom fruits and vegetables.

AVAILABILITY LEGEND

 Internet, Mail order   Locally   **R** Regionally   **S** Statewide

AISLE 1 GUIDE TO BRANDS

Company Logo	Contact/Corporate Information	Company Logo	Contact/Corporate Information

Berryluscious Farm
Gridley, CA 95948
530-846-3844
berryluscious.com

Frog Hollow Farm
Brentwood, CA 94513
888-779-4511
Independently Owned
froghollow.com

Bonipak Produce
Santa Maria, CA 93456
805-925-2505
bonipak.com

Homeless Garden Project
Santa Cruz, CA 95061
831-426-3609
CSA
homelessgardenproject.org

Bunny-Luv
Bakersfield, CA 93380
661-845-5200
Grimmway Farms
grimmway.com/bunnyluv

Kiva Orchards
Durango, CO 81302
970-259-2238
High Desert Foods
kivaorchard.com

Cascadian Farm
Sedro-Woolley, WA 98284
800-624-4123
Small Planet Foods
General Mills
cfarm.com

Long Wind Farm
East Thetford, VT 05043
802-785-4642
longwindfarm.com

CF Fresh
Sedro-Woolley, WA 98284
360-855-0566
cffresh.com

Made In Nature
Fowler, CA 93625
800-906-7426
madeinnature.com

Dole
Westlake Village, CA 91359
800-232-8888
Dole Foods, Inc.
Dole.com

Mariquita Farm
Watsonville, CA 95077
831-761-3226
mariquita.com

Earthbound Farm
San Juan Batista, CA 95405
800-690-3200
Natural Selection
Tanimura & Antle
ebfarm.com

Nojoqui Farm
Buellton, CA 93427
805-686-0194
Family owned
nojoquifarms.org

Echoes of Summer
West Chatham, MA 02669
262-763-9551
Family owned
echoesofsummer.com

Northern Lights Foods
La Ronge, SK S0J 1L0
306-425-3434
northernlightsfoods.com

AISLE 1 GUIDE TO BRANDS

Company Logo	Contact/Corporate Information	Company Logo	Contact/Corporate Information
PINE CREEK PACK NATURAL	**Pine Creek Pack** Omak, WA 98841 509-826-8003 Fruit grower coalition pinecreekpack.com		**Sweet Grass Farms** Kalispell, MT 59901 406-755-3711 sweetgrassfarms.com
	Sno-Pac Caledonia, MN 55921 800-533-2215 Family owned snopac.com	Uncle Matt's ORGANIC	**Uncle Matt's** Clermont, FL 34712 352-394-8737 unclematts.com
	Solana Gold Organics Sebastopol, CA 95473 800-459-1121 solanagold.com		**Willotta Ranch** Fairfield, CA 94534 707-864-0912 willottaranch.com
SOUTH TEX ORGANICS	**South Tex Organics** Mission, TX 78572 888-895-0108 Family owned stxorganics.com		**Willow Wind Organic Farms** Spokane, WA 99201 509-624-3700 willowwindfarms.com
	Swanton Berry Farm Davenport, CA 95017 831-469-8804 swantonberry.com 🅛	Wood Prairie	**Wood Prairie Farm** Bridgewater, ME 04735 800-829-9765 woodprairie.com

AISLE 2
Breads, Cereals, Pasta, and Grains

PROBABLY THE FIRST domesticated crops, grains—the staff of life—have provided the bulk of the human diet since the dawn of agriculture. Today half of the world's cultivated land grows some type of grain, translating into more than 75 percent of all the calories consumed by human beings. Noodles, breads, cereals, and rice make up an indispensable part of human nutrition, so how these essential grains are grown, milled, and processed has a profound impact on the health of individuals and the environment.

The term *grain* refers to any of a number of grasses whose seeds are, with some drying and processing, edible to humans. The two most important grain crops in the world are wheat and rice. Others include barley, oats, rye, and a whole host of "minor" grains. Although not technically grains, corn and soybeans are often lumped into this category because they grow in a manner similar to that of the major grains. But most of the corn and soybeans grown in the United States ends up as animal feed, corn syrup, and increasingly fuel. For that reason, corn and soybeans will be discussed here only insofar as their processed products become part of the human diet.

Organic grain production and processing follows much the same path as conventional, but some very important differences exist. In the next several pages, we will highlight these differences in order to help you decide whether buying organic grain products—baked goods, cereals, pastas, and rice—is a good way to spend your organic food dollar. Areas covered include:

- Wheat and minor grain production
- Rice production
- Problems with grains
- Corn and soybeans
- The organic difference
- Grain products

WHEAT AND MINOR GRAIN PRODUCTION

Since the earliest days of plant domestication, nearly every agricultural innovation along the way—from fertilizer to the plow—facilitated the growing of grain. Until about 1950, however, those innovations changed little. At the beginning of the twentieth century, grain production in the United States still resembled that of the Middle Ages. Real horsepower still tilled the soil, and farmers' own muscles scythed the crop. Using these methods on the average fifty-seven-acre farm[1] produced just twelve bushels of wheat per acre.[2] With the advent of tractors and combines, one farmer could handle more acres, but until the 1950s, the equipment did little to increase yields.

How did the yield of wheat manage to soar from twelve bushels per acre in 1900 to nearly forty-five today? A common misperception is that chemicals are the single source of increased production. The primary reason for this phenomenal growth in efficiency, however, is plant breeding.[3] Over the years wheat has been bred to produce more heads per plant, more kernels per head, and stronger, shorter stalks. In addition, wheat plants have been developed for greater resistance to drought and pests. Chemicals have also played a role in increased yields, although not to the extent some organic advocates lead consumers to believe.[4]

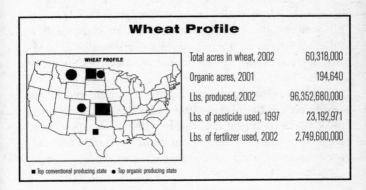

Wheat Profile

Total acres in wheat, 2002	60,318,000
Organic acres, 2001	194,640
Lbs. produced, 2002	96,352,680,000
Lbs. of pesticide used, 1997	23,192,971
Lbs. of fertilizer used, 2002	2,749,600,000

■ Top conventional producing state　● Top organic producing state

In addition to the pesticides and fertilizers, producers also use growth regulators. These plant hormones produce various effects, but the two most important for wheat are shortening the stem and getting the stem to branch. Shorter stems help keep the wheat from falling over. Encouraging the stem to branch produces more grain per plant. The natural growth regulators auxin, cytokinin, and gibberellins are allowed in organic production.

Although what has not escaped GEO tinkering, Monsanto's plans for Roundup Ready Wheat have been put on hold. A well-planned and executed campaign conducted by the Organic Consumers Association and others managed to convince both the domestic food industry and foreign buyers to boycott any introduction of GEO wheat.

Chemicals in Wheat Production

Conventional wheat production makes use of synthetic agricultural chemicals, whereas organic rules prohibit their use. Given the advantages to farming without synthetic chemicals, why isn't all wheat produced that way? The simple answer is that organic wheat production carries with it inherent problems in terms of scale of production. The efficiency achieved by conventional practices is difficult to match with organic methods.

While organic methods play an important role in the search for less harmful methods of production, the human health risks from pesticide residues on wheat appear to be slight. But problems with groundwater pollution from nitrates and herbicides remain (see Chapter 4).

Pest Problems in Storage

The use of chemicals in grain production doesn't end with the harvest. Once taken from the field, stored grain becomes vulnerable to destruction by pests—beginning at the regional grain elevators that dot the landscape of the Northern Plains. Here grain from area farms is pooled together awaiting transport to larger storage facilities and mills, where it will be converted into various flours for domestic use and export. Each stage presents problems with stored-grain pests.

Despite insecticides used in the field, grain carries with it the eggs and larvae of a whole host of insects. Killing eggs and larvae is not guaranteed even when the most potent pesticides are used on stored grain. It does not matter whether the grain is milled and further processed, grain-eating insects are everywhere in the production chain. Any grain product—whole, rolled, or flaked, pasta or flour—

will eventually become a feedlot for these exclamation-point-sized bugs.

Since *every* grain product is susceptible, conventional grains and flours are fumigated both in storage and in transit to ensure that the product does not exceed the FDA's bug parts-per-million limit. Organic grain relies on alternative bug-killing methods: "heat-ups,"* fumigations with carbon dioxide, biological controls, and many other less effective experimental methods. Organic products also rely on elaborate shipping schedules to ensure that consumers receive fresh, untainted supplies.

Shopping Tip

If you buy and store large quantities of pasta, flour, or cereal, you may experience the miracle of flour beetle eggs hatching. To avoid it, select packages with the latest sell-by date, particularly if it's a sale item. By discounting items with earlier dates, the store may be offering an incentive to alleviate its own potential bug problem. Finally, buy only an amount you can use within a month or two.

Grain Milling and Processing

Few grains are consumed as they are found in the field. All must undergo some processing, and several more steps

---

* A heat-up consists of raising the temperature of a mill or processing facility to the point where adult insects can no longer live. This method is complicated by the fact that excess heat often damages very expensive equipment. In addition, the cost of keeping large buildings at temperatures greater than 160 degrees is often prohibitive.

are necessary to create flour. First, the grain is cleaned to remove small stones, dirt, leaves, bugs, and other field debris. Screens, forced air, and magnets accomplish this task. Because organic grain is not treated with any fungicides, cleaning the grain is extremely important for reducing the chance of mold growth.

After cleaning, the grain must be dried so that its bran comes off in large pieces, a task accomplished with massive steel rollers that crush the grain into flour. Then it is sifted to separate the bran (its outer coating), the middlings (coarse-ground flour), the germ, and the flour. Although steel rollers are more efficient, health advocates claim that stone-ground whole wheat retains more nutrients because stone rollers do not overheat the grain.

Shopping Tip

The NOP's organic rule does not address the use of steel or stone mills, but several organic mills do use stones. If you purchase organic stone-ground wheat flour, be sure to store it under refrigeration, as it is prone to become rancid more quickly.

The initial stages of organic grain milling look much the same as those of conventional milling, but here is where the similarity ends. Conventional flour is processed with a number of chemicals designed to enhance bread making, storage life, appearance, and nutrition.

Natural aging makes wheat's gluten more elastic and promotes bread rising. To speed the process and artificially age conventional flour, potassium bromate is added to it. Critics of the baking industry claim that potassium bromate causes renal cancer in rats and thus should be prohibited in flour, as several European countries have done.

On the other hand, bread makers cite studies showing that manufacturing processes—bleaching, enriching, baking, and dough rising—eliminate potassium bromate residues from bread. The FDA's Total Diet Study confirms that no potassium bromate residues remain in bread. Conventional flour is also gassed with chlorine dioxide or benzoyl peroxide to change its natural yellowish color to white. Natural aging accomplishes the same process, and organic flour is allowed to age naturally.

As with raw grains, bugs make no distinction between organic and conventional flour. Organic mills rely on sanitation, alternative methods of pest control, and immediate shipping to control egg hatching. Conventional mills control bugs with chemical fumigation, which is prohibited in organic processing.

RICE PRODUCTION

Growing rice is very different from growing other grains, so what may hold true for most grains isn't necessarily so for rice. The United States produces about 25 billion pounds of rice per year on more than three million acres, mainly in Arkansas, Louisiana, and California. Conventional farmers frequently grow rice in water, not well-drained fertile soil. This production method presents different challenges for human and environmental health.

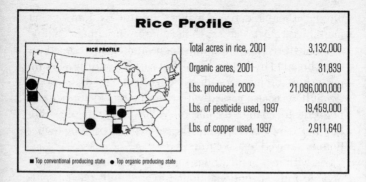

Rice Profile

Total acres in rice, 2001	3,132,000
Organic acres, 2001	31,839
Lbs. produced, 2002	21,096,000,000
Lbs. of pesticide used, 1997	19,459,000
Lbs. of copper used, 1997	2,911,640

■ Top conventional producing state ● Top organic producing state

First, water introduces a unique set of pests, such as tadpole shrimp and water weevils. Second, water supports a wide array of fungal diseases. Third, water supports abundant algae growth, a problem that most grain farmers in arid regions never even think about.

Conventional rice farmers turn to a substantial amount of chemicals to overcome these problems. Indeed, the rice grown in 2001 consumed nearly the same amount of pesticides as three times the amount of wheat. Some of these pesticides are unique and were developed solely for rice, while others may be used on other crops. For instance, four thousand times more fungicide was applied to rice than to wheat in 1997, but over 90 percent of that was copper, which is also approved for use in organic production.

Herbicides, as they do with many other crops, rank as the number-one pesticide used on rice—often applied directly to the standing water. Because herbicides in ground and surface water pose obvious problems, conventional rice production represents a greater threat to human health *via water contamination* than does wheat production.

Crop Rotation and Fertilization

In order to restore soil nutrients and alleviate problems with pests, both conventional and organic rice farmers rotate their crops. Conventional methods generally run on a simple, efficient two-year cycle of rice and soybeans. Organic practices employ a three- or four-year rotation of rice, soybeans, wheat, and fallow (growing nothing to rest the soil). Both conventional and organic farmers also use water to smother weeds, but organic methods—because they can't use synthetic pesticides—tend to drain fields sooner to flush the water-dependent pests out of the field.

All plants, like all people, require nutrients, and supplying agricultural crops with the nutrients they need poses perennial challenges. Conventional agriculture uses chemical fertilizers to augment crop rotation with soybeans. Without chemical fertilizers, organic rice production relies on green manure.* While more environmentally sound than using synthetic fertilizers, green manuring raises organic rice-production costs by twenty to thirty dollars per acre while producing 50 to 60 percent less than conventional rice.

PROBLEMS WITH GRAINS

Although the dietary risks associated with the chemicals used to produce grain are ambiguous, the environmental risks can be pinpointed and separated into two broad categories for most grains: soil compaction and erosion, and chemical contamination. (For rice, the risks are slightly different.)

---

* In the case of rice, soybeans are grown for their nitrogen-fixing capabilities, then plowed back into the soil.

Of all the agricultural commodities produced, grain uses the largest and heaviest equipment. This equipment bears responsibility for soil compaction, which in turn leads to chemical runoff, erosion, and reduction in yields. Although technological innovations in tires have lessened the problem, compaction correlates with the axle weight of the equipment. Both conventional and organic grain farms use cultivation and harvest equipment, but organic production relies on multiple cultivations to battle weed growth.

Grain production in the United States would not be economically feasible without this heavy equipment. In addition to soil compaction, frequent plowing and cultivation make soil vulnerable to both water and wind erosion. The following map details the relationship between growing regions and areas vulnerable to erosion.

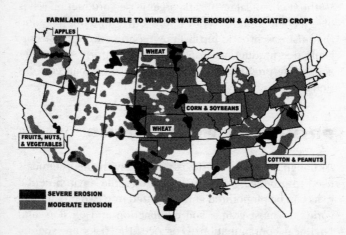

FARMLAND VULNERABLE TO WIND OR WATER EROSION & ASSOCIATED CROPS

Apart from rice, other conventional grains' production methods resemble those of wheat, except for the fact that substantially fewer chemicals are needed. In addition, most of the other grains grow in roughly the same geographical regions as wheat. Organic production methods, if widely employed, would reduce groundwater contamination but might do little to address erosion.

Rice production, even more than that of wheat and other grains, poses contamination problems for the environment: when water is drained from rice fields into local waterways, pesticides flow directly into surface waters. But the news isn't all bad. Researchers have found that the flooding of rice fields increases migratory waterfowl populations.

Another problem that accompanies conventional rice production is smoke. In order to reduce disease and insect pressures, conventional rice growers frequently set fire to their fields after harvest. The resulting emissions add greenhouse gases to the air, and the smoke has been known to reduce the visibility and cause accidents on California's Interstate 5. Residents repeatedly protest this practice, and the NOP rule addresses it, then provides a loophole. It says, "The producer must not use burning as a means of disposal for crop residues produced on the operation." However, "burning may be used to suppress the spread of disease or to stimulate seed germination."[5]

CORN AND SOYBEANS

Because corn and soybeans dominate conventional agriculture, we cannot consume conventional processed food without encountering them in some form. Moreover, they are the primary source of feed for much of the livestock in the United States. Of all commodities grown in this country, these crops consume the most fertilizers and much of the pesticide used in agriculture because they take up the majority of agricultural land. Corn and soybeans together cover more than 151 million acres—over 16 percent of all

U.S. farmland—primarily in the Midwest. Just seven states produce 70 percent of all the corn and soybeans grown in the United States. In fact, if all the corn and soybeans grown in one year were pooled together, it would fill 394 silos the size of the Empire State Building.

According to critics of modern farming, growing massive amounts of corn and soybeans is the equivalent of agricultural Armageddon. They often paint a picture in which midwestern farmers are under the total control of multinational corporations bent on forcing them to produce these two crops alone, while depleting the soil on millions of acres and threatening our health in the process. Critics state that corn growers become addicted to chemical applications and are committed to monocropping, reckless about energy use, oblivious to biodiversity issues, and insensitive to criticisms concerning genetically engineered crops.[6]

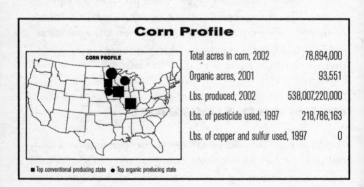

Corn Profile

Total acres in corn, 2002	78,894,000
Organic acres, 2001	93,551
Lbs. produced, 2002	538,007,220,000
Lbs. of pesticide used, 1997	218,786,163
Lbs. of copper and sulfur used, 1997	0

■ Top conventional producing state ● Top organic producing state

Growing Corn and Soybeans

First the good news: despite the perception, most conventional soybean and corn farmers retain control over how they farm. Contract growing makes up less than 20 percent of the corn and 10 percent of the soybeans produced. That said, large corporations still control most of the soybean and corn seed stock, machinery, and agricultural chemicals used to produce this bounty. But it is not true that the only seeds available are GEO varieties or that only a few seed companies control the supply. In 2003 the University of Minnesota's Extension Service tested 163 new varieties of soybeans from thirty-two different seed companies and/or research facilities. Twenty-five percent were not GEOs. Granted, this is not a large percentage, but it is perhaps more than one is led to believe by industrial agriculture's critics. Still, in the U.S. GEO varieties account for 80 percent of the soybean crop and nearly 50 percent of the corn crop.

Unfortunately, farmers still use nearly 32 billion pounds of chemical fertilizers and more than 300 million pounds of pesticides. Because 70 percent of this production takes place in just seven states, the groundwater of the Heartland continues to show heavy rates of contamination from herbicides and nitrates (see Chapter 4). The runoff from these fields ultimately ends up flowing down the Mississippi River into the Gulf of Mexico, severely damaging marine life. On the other hand, over 90 percent of the pesticides used are herbicides. As a result, very few residues show up in the corn or soybeans we eat—sort of a bad-for-groundwater, good-for-residues scenario. Of course, if you happen to live in the (rural) Midwest, herbicide runoff may directly affect your health as well.

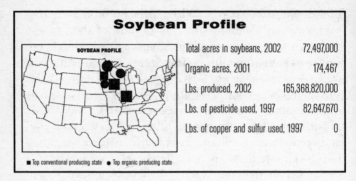

Soybean Profile

Total acres in soybeans, 2002	72,497,000
Organic acres, 2001	174,467
Lbs. produced, 2002	165,368,820,000
Lbs. of pesticide used, 1997	82,647,670
Lbs. of copper and sulfur used, 1997	0

▪ Top conventional producing state ● Top organic producing state

Between the 1880s and 1970s, farmers were often given merit badges for burying the most residues and tilling the straightest furrows, but current thinking now defines a tillage system by the amount of debris left standing in the field after harvest. Today corn and soybeans planted in midwestern fields employ one of three methods: conventional tillage, conservation tillage, or a combination of both.

Conservation tillage, which leaves anywhere from 30 to 100 percent of the previous crop on the field surface, benefits the environment by reducing not only soil erosion but also soil structure breakdown, disruption of the soil's microbes, loss of organic matter, soil compaction, and unnecessary fossil fuel use.

The upside is that corn and soybean farmers have managed during the last thirty years to lower the amount of total topsoil lost from 3.1 billion tons in 1982 to 1.91 billion tons in 1997 by using low-till methods with herbicides.[7] There is a trade-off, of course: groundwater contamination. Without herbicides, organic farmers must cultivate their fields, rotate crops, or plant cover crops in order to decrease weed pressure.

THE ORGANIC DIFFERENCE

Can corn and soybeans be grown successfully with organic production methods? The answer is a definite yes, although attention must be paid to corn's nitrogen needs. Intense green manure schedules, high organic matter from multiple plow-downs, and extensive crop rotation with soybeans can maintain a high level of nitrogen and good yields. Soybeans fit naturally into an organic rotation schedule.

The land devoted to organic corn production grew from 32,650 acres in 1995 to over 93,000 acres in 2001. Organic soybeans have done even better: from 47,200 to more than 174,000 acres in the same period. With the increase in organic meat, dairy, and soymilk consumption since 2001, this acreage has undoubtedly increased. Like their conventional counterparts, large organic producers also use corn and soybeans for the bulk of their feedstock—a limiting factor in the availability of organic dairy, eggs, poultry, and meat.

As industrial organic livestock production gears up to meet the demand, many traditional organic advocates fear that some benefits of organic production will be lost. Whereas most longtime organic farmers favor a five-to-six-year rotation schedule, conventional farmers converting to organic may find it easy to slip back into a two- or three-year rotation.

On top of that, the organic community, as production intensifies, must remain vigilant regarding the possibility of eroding standards, particularly when it comes to livestock. Organic soybean and corn prices are expected to remain high for several more years as conventional farms complete their three-year transitional phase. High prices encourage the exploitation of loopholes. In early 2003 an "organic" poultry producer in Georgia claimed that organic corn and soybeans for chicken feed were unavailable and sought legislative relief. Only the swift and vocal actions of the organic community managed to reverse the subsequent congressional attempt to lower standards.

The one obvious benefit of organic production is the elimination of the billions of pounds of chemicals used to produce conventional corn and soybeans. Today organic corn and soybean production covers less than a quarter of one percent of all lands growing these crops, and the number of organic acres needed to have a significant positive impact is unknown. But if organic sales continue to increase along the current trend lines of 20 percent annually through the year 2012, an additional 9.7 million total acres will need to come under organic production.[8] Corn and soybeans account for nearly 21 percent of all land growing organic crops. Consequently, a reasonable estimate for corn and soybean acreage growth is at least two million.

Forms and Availability of Grain

Grain	Available Organic	Flour	Coarse Ground	Whole Grain	Rolled	Bran	Cereal	Breads
Wheat	Yes	+++	+++	++	++	+++	+++	+++
Oats	Yes	++	++	++	+++	+++	+++	++
Corn	Yes	+++	+++	+++	+	+	+++	++
Rice	Yes	++	?	++++	?	?	+++	+
Rye	Yes	+++	+	?	+	+	?	+++
Kamut	Yes	++	+	+	?	?	++	++
Spelt	Yes	?	?	?	?	?	++	++
Triticale	Yes	++	+	+	?	?	?	+

Grain	Available Organic	Flour	Coarse Ground	Whole Grain	Rolled	Bran	Cereal	Breads
Quinoa	Yes	?	?	+++	+	+	?	?
Millet	Yes	++	?	++	?	?	?	?
Buckwheat	Yes	+++	?	++	?	?	+++	?
Amaranth	Yes	++	?	++	?	?	?	+
Sorghum	No	?	+	+	?	?	?	+
Barley & Malt	No	?	?	+++	+	+	?	?

Key: ? Availability unconfirmed, + Specialty, ++ Common, +++ Readily Available

GRAIN PRODUCTS

Even with the recent (waning) low-carb craze, products made from grain play a significant role in the American diet. The chart on the previous page and top of this page details the many different types of major and minor grains and the forms in which they may be found in our grocery stores.

Shopping Tip

Nutritionally, minor grains are comparable or superior to wheat, but bread made from them may not be as appealing. These other grains do, however, make delicious hot and cold cereals. The good news for shoppers seeking variety is that most of these unusual grains are grown organically.

Bread

Finding organic bread is easy. Several companies market it nationwide, and most areas have local alternative bakeries offering organic selections. As we discussed in

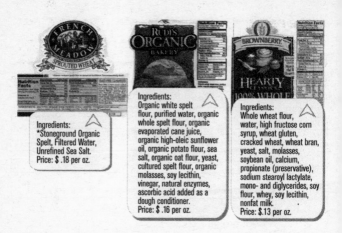

Ingredients:
*Stoneground Organic Spelt, Filtered Water, Unrefined Sea Salt.
Price: $ .18 per oz.

Ingredients:
Organic white spelt flour, purified water, organic whole spelt flour, organic evaporated cane juice, organic high-oleic sunflower oil, organic potato flour, sea salt, organic oat flour, yeast, cultured spelt flour, organic molasses, soy lecithin, vinegar, natural enzymes, ascorbic acid added as a dough conditioner.
Price: $ .16 per oz.

Ingredients:
Whole wheat flour, water, high fructose corn syrup, wheat gluten, cracked wheat, wheat bran, yeast, salt, molasses, soybean oil, calcium, propionate (preservative), sodium stearoyl lactylate, mono- and diglycerides, soy flour, whey, soy lecithin, nonfat milk.
Price: $.13 per oz.

Chapter 1, all bread labeled "organic" must have 95 to 100 percent of its ingredients produced organically. Most wheat and specialty grain breads easily meet this standard. But breads with herbs, cheese, seeds, or nuts are harder to produce organically. Breads (such as French Meadow's Men's and Women's Breads) formulated for specific health concerns—anticancer, longevity, or antioxidant—may be impossible to produce organically because specialty organic ingredients are either not available or are cost prohibitive.

Taste Check: Wheat Bread

We sampled two different kinds of organic bread available nationally and compared them with a popular conventional brand. One of the organic brands tasted almost exactly like its conventional counterpart, with a spongy sweetness; the other organic brand was more to our liking. In fact, the differences in taste and texture were so profound, it's really a different product entirely.

Cereal

Cereal processing runs down a slightly different path. Grains intended for hot cereals—conventional or organic—receive little processing beyond coarse grinding and have always been a good choice for breakfast nutrition.

Shopping Tip

Read the cereals' nutrition panels, and determine which selection is the healthiest for you and your family. Your investigation may yield surprising results—such as the fact that some conventional cereals are lower in salt, sugar, and fat than their organic counterparts. Remember, the "organic" label denotes only how ingredients were grown and processed—it doesn't necessarily mean they are nutritionally superior.

During the past decade, dozens of organic cold cereals have come on to the market. With ready-to-eat cold cereals, the trade-off for their convenience is the extra processing and added ingredients. You may wish to weigh your need for convenience with the fact that many cold cereals may not be the healthiest option for grain consumption.

Taste Check: Cold Cereal

We compared two popular oat cereals—one conventional and one organic—produced by the same parent company. In blind tests, we could not determine a difference. Other organic oat cereals had a mealier, grittier consistency that tended toward mushiness if eaten while reading the morning paper.

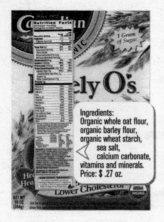

Ingredients:
Organic whole oat flour,
organic barley flour,
organic wheat starch,
sea salt,
calcium carbonate,
vitamins and minerals.
Price: $ .27 oz.

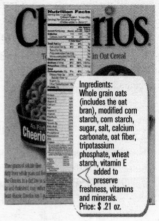

Ingredients:
Whole grain oats
(includes the oat
bran), modified corn
starch, corn starch,
sugar, salt, calcium
carbonate, oat fiber,
tripotassium
phosphate, wheat
starch, vitamin E
added to
preserve
freshness, vitamins
and minerals.
Price: $ .21 oz.

Pasta

During the last few years, the number of organic pasta choices escaped the confines of a slow boil. Twenty years ago you were lucky to find even conventional whole-wheat pasta, but today pasta is made from a variety of organic grains formed into bows, wiggles, wheels, and what-have-yous. While your local supermarkets may supply organic pasta in only a few forms (spaghetti or macaroni), natural food stores have devoted whole aisles to organic pasta.

BUYING GRAIN AND GRAIN-BASED FOODS

Whether you choose to spend your organic food dollar in the granary depends on your priorities. If pesticide residues concern you, the case for buying organic may be less compelling than for some fruits and vegetables. But an organic vote for these staple products may eventually lead to environmental relief for America's breadbasket. Wheat, corn, and soybeans can effectively be grown organically, and market pressures have already produced significant increases in acreage.

Best Bets

Grains	Number of Current Pesticide Residues	Number of Environmental Contaminants	Availability of Organic		Price Comparison Per Pound January '05	
			National Brands*	Local**	Organic	Conventional
✓Whole wheat bread***	10	2	W	W	$3.49	$1.922
White bread	18	6	L	L	$3.49	$2.10
Rye bread	14	6	W	L	$2.99	$1.69
Pasta	6	0	W	L	$2.59	$2.59
✓Rice, white	7	1	W	L	$2.99	$ .66
Oatmeal	9	1	W	L	$2.19	$ .99
Popcorn, in oil***	21	12	W	L	$ .89	$ .80

✓ = Best Bet for conventional

Source for Contaminants and Residues: FDA's Total Diet Study, 2002

* W = widely available; L = limited availability; H = hard to find; N/A = not available

** Seasonally available

*** These are residues found in processed products. Plain wheat flour was found to contain only two residues, while whole, unpopped corn had but one.

Grain Production Comparison: Conventional versus Organic

	Conventional	Organic
Fertilizer	Large amounts of nitrogen fertilizer use, resulting in significant groundwater contamination in grain country	High use of crop rotation, cover cropping, green manure, and compost
Pesticide Use	Heavy use of herbicides resulting in significant groundwater contamination in grain country; little pesticide residues on milled products	No use of herbicides or insecticides; mostly tractor cultivation and crop rotation for weed control
Post-Harvest Handling	Some stored grain products fumigated with phosphine; production facilities fumigated with methyl bromide, sulfury fluoride, or alternative methods	Alternative pest control methods used in all-organic operations; conventional methods used occasionally in split operations
Processing	Some chemicals used to process wheat into flour and bread; few chemicals used on rice or oat products	No chemicals used in grain processing

CONSUMER'S GUIDE

Aisle 2: Breads, Cereals, Pasta, and Grains

- Look for the USDA organic seal on all grain products.
- Avoid organic cold cereal products made with evaporated cane juice.
- Seek out organic *whole*-grain products.

- Seek out bread from local bakeries.
- Seek out grains and pasta from bulk bins.

- Seek out grain from farm co-ops supporting small grain farmers.

- Seek out artisan bread from local bakeries.

AVAILABILITY LEGEND

❶ Internet, Mail order ❶ Locally ❶ Regionally ❶ Statewide

AISLE 2 GUIDE TO BRANDS

Company Logo	Contact/Corporate Information	Company Logo	Contact/Corporate Information
	Alvarado Street Bakery Rohnert Park, CA 94928 707-585-3293 alvaradostreetbakery.com		**Breadshop** Boulder, CO 80301 800-434-4246 Hain-Celestial Heinz www.hain-celestial.com
	Ancient Harvest Gardena, CA 90248 310-530-8666 quinoa.net		**Cascadian Farm** Sedro-Woolley, WA 98284 800-624-4123 Small Planet Foods General Mills cfarm.com
	Annie's Homegrown Wakefield, MA 01880 781-224-1172 Annie's Homegrown, Inc. annies.com		**Country Choice** Eden Prairie, MN 55344 952-829-8824 countrychoicenaturals.com
	Arrowhead Mills Garden City, NY 11530 800-434-4246 Hain-Celestial Heinz arrowheadmills.com		**DaVinci Italian Organics** Paramus, NJ 07652 201-909-0808 InterNatural Foods internaturalfoods.com
	Back to Nature San Dimas, CA 91733 909-599-0961 Organic Milling Co. Kraft/Altria (Philip Morris) organicmilling.com		**DeBoles** Boulder, CO 80301 800-434-4246 Hain-Celestial Heinz www.hain-celestial.com
	Barbara's Bakery Petaluma, CA 94954 707-765-2273 barbarasbakery.com		**Eden Foods** Clinton, MI 49236 888-424-EDEN Independently owned eden-foods.com
	Bella Terra (Racconto) Melrose Park, IL 60161 racconto.com		**Envirokidz** Blaine, WA 98230 604-248-8777 Nature's Path Foods envirokidz.com
	Bob's Red Mill Milwaukie, OR 97222 800-553-2258 Bob's Red Mill Natural Foods bobsredmill.com		**Erewhon** Needham, MA 02494 800-422-1125 U.S. Mills usmillsinc.com

AISLE 2 GUIDE TO BRANDS

Company Logo	Contact/Corporate Information	Company Logo	Contact/Corporate Information

Familia
Paramus, NJ 07652
201-909-0808
InterNatural Foods
internaturalfoods.com

Fiddler's Green Farm
Belfast, ME 04915
800-729-7935
Family owned
fiddlersgreenfarm.com

Food For Life Baking Co.
Corona, CA 92878
909-279-5090
foodforlife.com

French Meadow
Minneapolis, MN 55408
877-669-3278
Independently owned
frenchmeadow.com

Gold Medal Organic
Minneapolis, MN 55440
800-328-1144
General Mills
generalmills.com

Golden Temple
800-225-3623
goldentemple.com

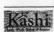

Kashi Company
La Jolla, CA 92039-8557
858-274-8870
Kellogg
kashi.com

Lowell Farms
El Campo, TX 77437
979-543-4950
lowellfarms.com

Lundberg Family Farm
Richvale, CA 95974
530-882-4551
Family owned
lundberg.com

Natural Value
Sacramento, CA 95831
916-427-7242
Family owned
naturalvalue.com

Nature's Organic Goodness
Barrie, ONT L4N 8Z6
800-353-3178

Nature's Path
Vancouver, BC
888-808-9505
Family owned
naturespath.com

Odwalla
Half Moon Bay, CA 94019
800-ODWALLA
Minute Maid
Coca-Cola
odwalla.com

Olio Beato
Scarsdale, NY 10583
914-723-5850
Pietro DeMarco Importers
organicoil.com

Oregon Chai
Portland, OR 97209
888-874-2424
oregonchai.com

Organic Classics
Brockton, MA 02301
877-400-5997
Fairfield Farm Kitchens
fairfieldfarmkitchens.com

AISLE 2 GUIDE TO BRANDS

Company Logo	Contact/Corporate Information	Company Logo	Contact/Corporate Information
Organic Coffee Co.	**Organic Coffee Co.** San Leandro, CA 94577 510-638-1300 o-coffee.com **S**	**Pastorelli**	**Pastorelli** Chicago, IL 60607 800-767-2829 pastorelli.com
	Organic Cow of Vermont Tunbridge, VT 05077 888-490-3020 Horizon Dean Foods horizonorganic.com/theorganiccow **R**		**Paul's Grains** Laurel, IA 50141 641-476-3373 Family owned paulsgrains.com **O**
Organic Gourmet	**Organic Gourmet** Sherman Oaks, CA 91403 800-400-7772 organic-gourmet.com	**PEACE CEREAL**	**Peace Cereal** Eugene, OR 800-225-3623 Golden Temple peacecereal.com **S**
	Organic Planet Philadelphia, PA 19119 215-753-7171 organicplanet.com **O**	**RISING MOON ORGANICS**	**Rising Moon Organics** Eugene, OR 97402 541-431-0505 risingmoon.com
Organic Valley	**Organic Valley** La Farge, WI 54693 888-444-6455 Farmer owned co-op—CROPP organicvalley.com	**Rudi's ORGANIC**	**Rudi's** Boulder, CO 80301 877-293-0876 Rudi's Organic Bakery rudisbakery.com
	Organic Vintners Importers Boulder, CO 80302 303-245-8773 organicvintners.com **O**	Shiloh Farms	**Shiloh Farms Bakery** Sulphur Springs, AR 72768 479-298-3297 users.nwark.com/~shilohf/ **O**
	Our Family Farm Newport, KY 41071 859-261-2627 Family owned ourfamilyfarm.com	SONORA MILLS	**Sonora Mills Foods** Rancho Dominguez, CA 90221 310-639-5333 sonoramills.com
Pamela's	**Pamela's Products** San Francisco, CA 650-952-4546 pamelasproducts.com **O**	Southern BROWN RICE	**Southern Brown Rice** Weiner, AR 72479 800-421-7423 southernbrownrice.com

AISLE 2 GUIDE TO BRANDS

Company Logo	Contact/Corporate Information	Company Logo	Contact/Corporate Information

Stephanie's Bakery
San Diego, CA 92107
619-221-0285
stephaniesbakery.com

Vita Spelt
Okemos, MI 48864
517-351-9231
Purity Foods
purityfoods.com

Sweet Wheat

Sweet Wheat
Clearwater, FL 33757
727-442-5454
sweetwheat.com

Vital Vittles
Berkeley, CA 94710
510-644-2022
vitalvittles.com

Sylvan Border Farm
Willits, CA
707-459-1854
sylvanborderfarm.com

Weetabix.

Weetabix
Clinton, MA 01510
978-368-0991
weetabixusa.com

Tumaro's
Los Angeles, CA 90029
323-464-6317
tumaros.com

Wholly Healthy

Wholly Healthy
Morristown, NJ 07962
800-247-6580
whollyhealthy.com

AISLE 3
Seeds, Beans, Nuts, and Oils

BOTANICALLY SPEAKING, there is no difference between a seed, a bean, a nut, and a grain. They are all seeds. Culturally, however, a seed with a hard shell is a nut; a seed that requires milling is a grain; and a seed from a legume is a bean. Whether we are cracking peanuts at a ballgame or drizzling oil and vinegar over a plate of greens, we tend to overlook the humble seed and pay scant attention to the versatility and ubiquity of seeds in our diets.

With a wary public concerned about the potential health effects of meat consumption, nuts and beans have become increasingly popular as alternative sources of protein and fiber. Even when seeds, nuts, and beans are not eaten directly, their high fat content has made the oils derived from them an integral part of modern food processing and preparation. In 1997, for example, Americans consumed over eight billion pounds of oil derived from seeds.[1] Clearly, seeds are not just for the birds.

This Aisle will explore the varied roles seeds play in our diets, outlining some of the differences in the production of:

- Seeds
- Beans
- Nuts and nut butters
- Oils

SEEDS

Although we may not immediately think of seeds as an important part of our diet, they play crucial roles at mealtime. As spices, oils, or whole, seeds enhance salads and sandwiches. Without oil, some cooking and baking methods would not be possible. Some seeds, such as sesame and sunflower, make fine oils as well as spices and garnishes. Others, like canola and safflower, enter our diets only as oil. The following chart lists available seeds and their uses. Organic versions can be found for all.

Seed Uses and Organic Availability

Seeds	Uses	Organic Available?
Sesame, sunflower	whole, oil, butter	yes
Pumpkin	whole, raw, roasted	yes
Canola (rapeseed), safflower	oil	yes
Flax	whole, meal, oil	yes
Mustard, caraway, cumin, poppy, celery, anise, dill, coriander, fennel	spices	most
Alfalfa, broccoli, radish, fenugreek, kale, lentils, mustard, onion, sunflower, wheat	sprouts	most

A Seed Sown

Most seed crops grow in rows, subject to the same threats as other agricultural commodities. Each has specific requirements that dictate where and how it is grown. Canola seeds grow well in Canada's short season, and safflower and sunflower do just fine in North Dakota. Other seeds, such as sesame, are imported from Mexico. Seeds for direct consumption lend themselves to small local producers, while oil seeds come from larger acreages. For big organic growers, oil seeds often earn a place in a five- to six-year rotation plan. Conventional farms seldom extend their rotations beyond three different crops.

BEANS

Beans can be placed into three categories based on their geographical region of origin: New World, Old World, and Asian. As late as 1977, most Americans were acquainted only with peas and New World beans, and the average American consumed just over six pounds of dry edible beans per year. But as ethnic and fusion cuisines expanded beyond community borders, Old World and Asian legume consumption increased, bringing the total to eight and a half pounds per person in 1997.[2]

The Incredible, Edible Soybean

Until the 1960s soybeans were a minor crop grown under the radar of the average U.S. consumer. In 1917, for example, U.S. farmers planted fewer than half a million acres. Today 76 million acres of soybeans cover vast swaths of the Midwest. Domesticated in China more than five thousand years ago, the soybean's versatility makes it an essential part of America's modern agricultural economy, providing a source of protein for cows, pigs, and chickens. In addition, these multitalented legumes have become an important element in both the alternative fuel and pharmaceutical industries.

As a part of the human diet, soy products and ingredients have become ubiquitous in the modern food supply, despite the fact that most Americans don't eat them the way they might prepare pinto or navy beans. Plain cooked soybeans just don't taste very good, but they can seemingly be made into anything, from milk to meatless "bacon." Tofu, tempeh, miso, and natto have now joined soy sauce as familiar and widely available soy foods. With their many uses, soybeans have had a dramatic impact on the U.S. food supply in the last two decades.

Bean Production

Beans have a lot going for them. Nutritionally, they provide fiber and protein. Agriculturally, they grow well in a variety of climates and serve the vital purpose of building soil nutrients. Nearly every region of the country produces dry edible beans, but arid climates make up the highest production areas because of the reduced pest and disease impact.

Because dry beans are legumes, they perform the miracle of taking nitrogen from the air and turning it into a usable plant nutrient. Both conventional and organic farmers take advantage of this fact by planting beans in rotation with wheat, corn, and other crops. The ability to fix nitrogen means that they require little, if any, nitrogen fertilizer, but conventional farmers usually apply synthetic phosphorus and potassium at planting time. Organic growers often apply rock-bearing minerals to supply these nutrients.

Bacteria and the Beanstalk

All farmers, conventional and organic, inoculate bean seeds before planting them. Inoculation involves coating the seed with various rhizobacteria strains. These bacteria aid in the nitrogen-fixing process by forming nitrogen-filled nodules on the plants' roots. After harvesting the crop, these nodules are left behind to fertilize the soil. Rhizobacteria are natural residents of the soil, but seed treatments enhance their benefits to both bean and soil.

Each legume (peas, clover, peanuts, etc.) requires its own kind of rhizobacteria, so laboratories grow different strains in large vats and label each inoculant according to its legume partner. Farmers mix the proper inoculants with the seeds before planting. Because the bacteria used in conventional production are now genetically engineered, NOP regulations require that all inoculants for organic production be GEO free.

Pests and Beans: Are Pesticides a Problem?

Bean plants' small stature puts them at a disadvantage when competing with weeds, so conventional farmers rely on both cultivation and herbicides to combat plant pests. Most conventional farmers till weeds first, then switch to herbicides later in the season. Organic producers control weeds through crop rotation and tillage, although neither method provides complete relief. Consequently, organic beans may suffer higher yield losses.

Insects bother beans, but not to the extent of other crops. Conventional farmers use dicofol—by far the most heavily applied insecticide—to control fast-breeding mites that can become a serious problem very quickly. Recently, conventional farmers have become more reliant on integrated pest management (IPM), scouting their fields and spraying insecticides only when an economic threshold is reached. Large organic growers use insecticides allowed by the NOP, such as garlic, neem, natural pyrethrum, and diatomaceous earth.

Beans may succumb not only to weeds and bugs but

also to fungal diseases. Although many varieties grow in arid climates, extended periods of wet weather may trigger either fungal or bacterial diseases. Conventional as well as organic growers use both copper and sulfur to combat fungus. Although conventional farmers have a larger arsenal of chemicals at their disposal, many still place a high priority on crop rotation. In a sense, they move the crop away from the problem rather than spraying the problem away. Organic farmers, too, rely on rotating crops into clean fields. They also create buffer zones that harbor beneficial insects, and they till-in green manures to improve the soil's organic matter. As for pesticide residues, in 2001 the USDA tested for 130 chemical residues in twenty-four samples of various dry beans and found no residues.

Harvesting, Cleaning, and Storage

Traditionally, beans were allowed to dry completely in the field, but modern conventional bean growers use sodium chlorate to wither the leaves and lower the moisture in the beans before they harvest them. Wet leaves hamper the harvest, and damp beans invite dangerous mold to grow in storage. Organic farms rely on grain-drying units to control the moisture after harvest, but crop drying requires a lot of energy use on both organic and conventional farms.

All beans are cleaned using forced air and sifting to remove foreign material (straw, chaff, weed seeds, soil, small pebbles, and dead insects). Cleaning extends the storage life, reduces damage done by disease, and ultimately improves the yield. Organic bean-cleaning facilities must be certified and undergo annual inspections.

Buying Beans

Dry beans sold in supermarkets usually come in one-pound plastic bags. In food co-ops and natural food chains, they may also be available in more economical bulk bins (the least expensive option). For the consumer seeking convenience, organic beans are now offered precooked and canned, as well.

The question of organic and conventional beans' relative worth is, as with many other products, a question about priorities and concerns. If pesticide residues on edible beans are your only worry, you may consider spending your money on conventional beans—testing rarely documents any residues. *But if you are concerned with biotechnology's effect on health or the environment, then soybeans and their products pose a problem. Over 85 percent of conventional soybeans raised in the United States are genetically engineered.*

NUTS AND NUT BUTTERS

Nuts have long enjoyed a nutritious image, finding their way into many of the original "health foods": trail mix, nut butters, granola, and energy bars. In their role as seeds, they contain all the valuable nutrients a plant needs to grow, and we omnivores figured out long ago how to capitalize on this fact. High in both protein and fat, nuts supply a compact source of energy in natural packaging. For the most part, their fat content is comprised of both unsaturated and monosaturated fats, otherwise known as the "good" fats. They are also high in vitamins and fiber.

Nut Production

Tree nuts are a perennial crop grown in orchards in the same manner as tree fruits. Of the 2.3 billion-pound domestic nut crop (mostly almonds, pistachios, and walnuts), California produces 73 percent. As with other conventional crops grown in California, critics of conventional nut production claim it is unsound for the environment and poses risks to our health.

Pesticides and Tree Nuts

Industrial agriculture proponents claim that the hard shells of nuts protect them from pesticides, and that nut farms use no more chemicals than any other kind of farms. Actually, almonds use slightly higher amounts per pound produced than many of the produce items covered in Aisle 1, but residues do not pose a significant problem for almonds and other shelled nuts. Both the industry and its critics are correct.

In addition, more than half of all the pesticides used on almonds are the same chemicals allowed for use in organic almond production. *Nuts are another case where if you are buying organic tree nuts solely out of fear of pesticide residues, your money could be better spent elsewhere. If, however, you are committed to buying organic because of a concern for the environment and the human beings who grow and harvest nuts, then your money will be well spent on organic nuts.*

Peanuts

Nuts do not just grow on trees. The ever-popular peanut is actually the seed of a legume, not a tree, and grows underground. Planted in the early spring primarily in

Georgia, Arkansas, and Texas, conventional peanut farmers usually include them in a three-year rotation with cotton, corn, sorghum, or soybeans.

After the plant flowers and pollinates, peanuts form underground and must be harvested by digging. They are left to dry in the field several days before being raked up and hauled to a buying station. In some cases, forced air may be applied to further dry the peanuts—a crucial step because it reduces the chances of mold. The remaining peanut vines, and their pesticide residues, become bales of animal fodder.

Once at the buying station, USDA officials grade the peanuts and inspect them for *Aspergillus flavus* mold. Its waste product, aflatoxin, can be acutely poisonous when high levels are consumed and carcinogenic when consumed regularly at low levels (see Chapter 3).

Pesticides and Peanuts

In addition to the poisonous aflatoxin mold, peanuts have other pest-related problems. Before planting, conventional farmers inject a fumigant called metam sodium into the soil to prevent "black rot," a common peanut ailment, and to combat nematodes and fungi. Although there are health risks to exposed farm workers and wildlife during application, the fumigant does not show up as a residue in peanuts.

The number of other chemical residues found on peanuts fell during the past decade. In 1997, 28 percent of peanut samples contained some residues. By 2002,* only 18 percent revealed residues, reflecting both the use of less persistent pesticides and better integrated pest management systems.

---

* The USDA's Pesticide Data Program does not test every food commodity every year. Many crops are only periodically tested.

Regrettably, residues that do show up in peanut products are disturbing. Health Canada (the Canadian FDA) also conducts a Total Diet Study* that showed long-banned insecticides and their breakdown products in peanuts and peanut butter. The high concentrations of lindane metabolites like HCH raise particular concern. The U.S. Department of Health and Human Services considers HCH a potential carcinogen in humans. Organic production methods are not immune to these types of persistent residues.

Nut Butters

In addition to playing key roles at ballparks, bars, and bridge tables, peanuts are churned into over 500 million pounds of peanut butter each year. One company manages to crank out 250,000 jars every day.[3] As far back as the 1920s, food faddists claimed one could find true health by consuming nothing but fruit and freshly made peanut butter. Today peanut butter is still a highly regarded, popular product touted as a good source of protein and vitamins.

Shopping Tip

The real difference between organic nut butters and their conventional counterparts can be found in the final grinding stage—where sugar, salt, and "partially hydrogenated" oils are added. The addition of hydrogenated oil keeps the peanut oil from separating and floating to the top, but these additional oils introduce trans-fatty acids into the final product. Most organic peanut butters do not add hydrogenated vegetable oils or sweeteners.

---

* For some reason, Health Canada chooses to publish residue results in everyday English as opposed to the FDA, whose results require the reader to have a background in chemistry.

While conventional and organic peanut butter production both involve the same steps—roasting, shelling, deskinning, screening, and grinding—the organic versions tend to be more "pure" (see Taste Check).

Taste Check: Peanut Butter

We compared a popular organic peanut butter to a conventional counterpart. The familiar creaminess and smooth mouthfeel of conventional peanut butter gave way to a stickier, nuttier flavor in the organic butter. Essentially, these are two different products. The organic version contains ground peanuts; conventional butters contain other ingredients added to achieve the taste and texture to which most consumers have become accustomed.

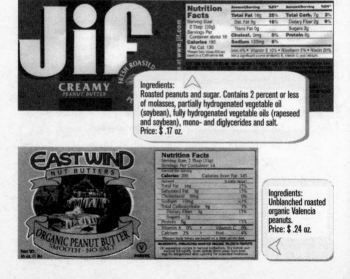

Ingredients:
Roasted peanuts and sugar. Contains 2 percent or less of molasses, partially hydrogenated vegetable oil (soybean), fully hydrogenated vegetable oils (rapeseed and soybean), mono- and diglycerides and salt.
Price: $ .17 oz.

Ingredients:
Unblanched roasted organic Valencia peanuts.
Price: $ .24 oz.

OILS

McDonald's makes billions of dollars selling it. Julia Child insisted it made food taste better. And Dr. Atkins promoted it like a used car salesman. In the end, paraphrasing Ms. Sara Lee just about sums it up: "Nobody doesn't like fat." Of course, there is another side to the story: eating fat contributes to high cholesterol, obesity, heart disease, and strokes.

People have been squeezing oil from seeds and certain fruits for thousands of years. Throughout history the oil press—with its large stone wheel—was a common sight. Modern food processing, however, has managed to turn a simple operation into an intense and complicated process. The reasons for this complication are both plant and profit related.

Organic Oils: Uses and Availability

Source	Saturated Fat	Omega-3 Fatty Acids*	Uses	Organic Available?**
Almond	7%	L	dessert salads, body care	yes
Apricot kernel	N/A	H	dessert salads, body care	in products
Avocado	17%	L	salads, condiments	yes
Canola	7%	H	salads, frying, baking	yes
Coconut	92%	L	candy, cookies, margarine, soaps	yes
Corn	13%	M	frying, salads, margarine	yes
Flaxseed	7%	H	nutritional supplements, condiments, salads	yes
Grapeseed	10%	L	sautéing, frying, salads	yes

Organic Oils (Continued)

Source	Saturated Fat	Omega-3 Fatty Acids*	Uses	Organic Available?**
Hazelnut	7%	M	baking, sauces, broiling, body care	yes
Hemp	10%	H	nutritional supplements, body care	in products
Lemon oil	N/A	N/A	desserts, condiments	in products
Macadamia	13%	M	body care, nutritional supplements	in products
Olive	14%	M	condiments, salads	yes
Palm fruit	52%	L	ethnic cooking, processed foods	in products, shortening
Palm kernel	86%	L	margarine, processed foods	in products
Peanut	18%	L	deep fat frying	yes
Pine nut	N/A	N/A	condiments	unknown
Pumpkin seed	15%	M	condiments, salads	yes
Rice bran	26%	M	frying, sautéing, body care	in body care products
Safflower	7%	L	frying, salads, processed foods	yes
Soybean	15%	M	baked goods, margarine, processed foods	yes
Sesame	15%	L	condiments, Asian foods	yes
Sunflower	15%	L	frying, salads, candy, processed foods	yes
Tea	10%	M	condiments, Asian foods, body care	in body care products

Organic Oils (Continued)

Source	Saturated Fat	Omega-3 Fatty Acids*	Uses	Organic Available?**
Walnut	9%	H	salads, sauces	yes
Wheat germ	17%	M	nutritional supplements, condiments, salads	yes

* H= high; M=medium; L=low

** "In products" means the oil is difficult to find in an organic form for the home cook.

Seed and fruit oils have long been a subject of contention among health advocates. Aside from the creative blending and renaming of different oilseeds for processed products (see sidebar below and on the next page), the only new twist in the saga is that the word *organic* now appears on the ever-burgeoning list of oily buzzwords. Is there a real difference between organic, unrefined oil and a bottle of Wesson?

By Any Other Name . . .

Canola oil is a relative newcomer to the cooking oil pantheon. It began to appear on grocers' shelves in the 1980s and soon attracted attention from health-conscious consumers because it is high in omega-3 fatty acids. But canola's origin is Asian, and India has been pressing *Brassica napus L.* seeds into oil for centuries. Unfortunately, its common name is not very flattering: rapeseed.

Rapeseed is a hardy annual in the mustard family* and

---

* The *Brassicaceae* family includes other well-known members: cabbage, cauliflower, and broccoli.

as such can be grown in areas with short, cool growing seasons—which is why the Canadian government started researching it as a potential crop back in the 1950s. Although rapeseed fits Canada's climate like a winter mitten, its name had to be overhauled. Voila! Canola—from CANada plus OIL—was christened.

Some media information suggests that canola seed is a different species from rapeseed. Not true, but since its introduction it has undergone hybridization, including genetic engineering. While Canada is the leading producer of canola seeds for oil, North Dakota also produces impressive amounts.

Oil Production

Oil production can be broken down into three basic steps: pre-extraction, extraction, and refining. Each of these large steps contains a number of subprocesses that—save one—are allowed in organic production. Whether the oil is produced from seeds, nuts, or beans the processes are similar, although not all of the steps pertain to oil-bearing seeds and fruits.

Pre-Extraction and Extraction. As its name suggests, this step prepares raw beans for their future incarnation as oil by cleaning, cracking, dehulling, separating, steaming, and rolling the beans into flakes.

The flaky mash then heads for the extraction process. Three methods are used commercially. The first, *hydraulic pressing,* squeezes the flakes between heavy metal plates. Because this method works best for crops with high oil content—sesame seeds and olives—it is not generally applied to large-scale oil production.

Expeller pressing uses a large cylindrical container with porous sides fitted with a spiral-shaped auger. The material is fed in at one end while the auger turns and presses the material against the sides, expelling the oil through the pores. The action of this screw press generates heat, and the oil can reach temperatures as high as 275°F. Some expeller presses are fitted with refrigerated tubes to cool the oil. Although the National Organic Standards Board has recommended that oil be "mechanically pressed (expeller pressed), hydraulic pressed, or stone pressed,"[4] the NOP rule did not single out any particular process for use in organic production. Most organic oil-processing plants use the expeller press method.

While producers sometimes use expeller presses, today *solvent extraction* remains the most commonly employed conventional method. This process involves placing the cooked and flaked bean material on a perforated plate or screen, then pumping hexane over it.* The hexane percolates down through the material, creating a soupy mush called miscella. An evaporator separates the hexane from the crude oil, and the de-oiled solid matter is pressed and molded into seed cake for use in animal feed. Solvent extraction is not allowed in organics, and solvent-extracted seed cake cannot be used in organic feed.

Finishing School. The final stage of oil production turns crude oil into the familiar products you see on grocery shelves. Refining oil is a bit more complicated than just running it through a filter. Included in this stage of production are degumming (the part of the process that yields the food additive lecithin), adding caustic soda with heat, bleaching, hydrogenating, deodorizing, and winterizing. All

---

* Hexane is the most frequently used solvent. Other solvents include pentane, heptane, trichloroethylene, and octane.

of the aforementioned processes (except adding solvents) are allowed in organic production, despite some concerns.

Any food-production process that involves heating (almost all do) tends to destroy some of the nutrients—an underlying reason for the marketing of "cold-pressed" oils. In seed oil production, a mix of sodium hydroxide and crude oil is heated to 200 degrees, then centrifuged to remove free fatty acids and other unwanted materials. This step is not prohibited in organic production.

Bleaching is another point of contention. Because U.S. consumers prefer lighter oils, conventional processors use fuller's earth* or activated charcoal in a vacuum—both of which are prohibited in organic processing. Organic processors filter their oil through natural clays such as bentonite or kaolin to absorb color pigments from the oil. Crude oil eventually slated for salad oil or margarine is not bleached extensively because it can remain yellow, but oil destined to become shortening is bleached even further.

Hydrogenation—the process that allows oil to become solid at room temperature—is the most problematic process in oil refining. Even liquid oil, particularly soybean, undergoes at least partial hydrogenation, which increases the oil's smoking point (for cooking purposes) and improves its shelf life. Unfortunately, this molecular musical-chairs game also changes both organic and conventional oils' healthy component—omega-3 fatty acids—into the undesirable *trans-fatty acids* partly responsible for cardiovascular disease.[5]

The last two processes, deodorization and winterization, remove sharp flavors and odors to create bland, relatively tasteless, and pure-looking oil suitable for cooking. Again,

---

* Fuller's earth is a clay consisting of aluminum, silica, iron oxides, lime, and magnesium. It is prohibited for use in organic production, as is charcoal.

these processes involve both heating and cooling the oil. Both are allowed in organic production.

Pesticides in Oil

Just as pesticides tend to migrate to the fat cells of animals, they also show up in plant oils. In the FDA's Total Diet Study, both conventional olive oil and safflower oil showed some chemical contaminates—most frequently DDT, endosulfan, and other contaminants from processing, transportation, and plastic packaging.[6] Organic oils were not tested, but organic production rules do not offer protection from these particular contaminants.

FATS AND PESTICIDES

The topic of fat is everywhere these days—in our newspapers, magazines, and diet books. It's on our TVs, radios, and computers. Mostly, however, fat is on our thighs, hips, and tummies, in what is called *adipose tissue.* The cells in this tissue serve as the body's storage lockers—excess calories are stored as fat. All plants and animals use this method of dealing with stuff their bodies can't break down.

Unfortunately, adipose tissue welcomes other things our bodies don't use, such as the chemical contaminants we consume with every meal—not just from pesticides, but also from indoor and outdoor air pollution, packaging, and cleaning solvents.

Any discussion about pesticide residues in organic food must confront this issue. Many of the chemicals that accumulate in our fat cells come from long-banned, persistent environmental contaminants. Although few organic fats and oils have been tested, there is no reason to believe they would be immune to these particular types of chemicals.

Despite NOP regulations regarding synthetic chemical inputs, their existence in our world is a fact of modern life. While several studies indicate that organic farming can reduce the residues from currently used synthetic pesticides, there is no evidence that organic food can protect us against the chemicals that persist in the environment.

Palm Oil

A recent trend in processed organic products is the use of organic palm oil. Given the dubious reputation of the highly saturated tropical oils, why would organic cookie makers highlight palm oil in their marketing? According to the package of Newman's Own Chocolate Crème Filled Cookies, the oil from the kernel is highly saturated, while the oil from the fruit is less so.[7] Manufacturers tout palm fruit oil as cancer preventing, loaded with vitamin A, and heart healthy—despite the fact that it is 50 percent saturated.

Organic palm fruit oil does allow processors to produce look-alike versions of the snack foods Americans crave. It may make crackers crispy, cookies crunchy, icings creamy, and cakes moist. It may also be an example of another food industry bill of goods.

Olive Oil

Americans have only recently discovered the wonders of olive oil, which is at least one reason you've never seen Popeye putting it on his spinach. Until olive oil slipped into the mainstream during the 1980s, ethnic communities accounted for most U.S. consumption. In 1982 the United States imported just 83 million pounds of it, but by 1998 366 million pounds came ashore.

Although the number of both conventional and organic

olive growers in California has climbed during the last two decades, domestic production still accounts for *less than 1 percent* of all the olive oil consumed in the United States. While much of this oil is "made in Italy," the olives are often grown in Turkey, Syria, and Tunisia. What is true for conventional is true for organic: most olive production lies outside the United States.

Growing Olives. Olives, like any other tree fruit, grow in orchards, but compared to other orchard crops, fewer *synthetic* chemicals are used in conventional production. In fact, 66 percent of all pesticides used on olives are the same as those approved for organic production.

Pressing Concerns. Because olives are high in oil, it can be easily extracted. In fact, Greek and Italian peasants often crushed olives as they did grapes— with their feet. Images of slaves pushing stone oil wheels abound in Roman frescoes.

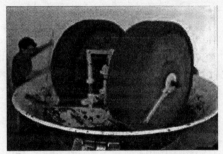

Source: Apollo Oil Co.

Today a few small producers still use a stone press.

As olives are pressed, the oil first released is considered the best quality. The pressed olives, called *pomace,* are milled several times to extract all the oil. The final pressing usually yields *lampante,* which roughly translates to "lamp oil."

Since the use of olive oil is still new to many Americans, it manages to maintain a certain mystique. Oil merchants have capitalized on this with what can be called "olive oil dogma." Many consumers remain confused by the labels "virgin" and "extra-virgin" oil.* Shoppers get the impression that *extra-virgin* means oil from the first pressing (which may or may not be true). The olive oil industry, on the other hand, uses the term *virgin* to indicate the level of acidity. Extra-virgin is defined as having less than 1 percent acid. Other terms are superfine virgin (1.10 to 1.50 percent acid); fine virgin (1.51 to 3.00 percent); virgin (3.10 to 4.00 percent); and lampante (4.10 to 5.00 percent).

Extra-virgin olive oil is often made with a stone, hydraulic, or expeller press. In many instances, virgin oil, as listed above, is from a third or fourth pressing. The lamp oil that is made today—obtained through solvent extraction after all the edible oil has been removed—is not actually used in lamps but is sold for industrial purposes.

Buying Oil

While small label, gourmet olive oils abound, finding other kinds of *organic* oil in some markets can be a bit of a chore, but several brands offer it. The exception is Spectrum Naturals, which can usually be found in any conventional supermarket that carries a limited selection of organic products.

As with many processed foods, few qualities separate organic and conventional oils. Incorporating the healthiest oil into your diet may take some adjustment. The best choice is unrefined oil that has not been processed with nutrition-reducing high heat. All pressing adds some heat from the friction, but expeller presses equipped with refrigerated tubing remedy this problem. The trick is to find a manufacturer that clearly states on the label that *refrigerated*

---

* *Virgin* is a term applicable only to olive oil, so other oil labels making that claim do so erroneously.

expeller presses are used. The label "cold-press" has no legal meaning and is not an indication that the bean, seed, or nut from which the oil has been made has been grown organically.

As for unrefined oils, most have strong flavors and cannot be used for high-temperature frying, but they may be acceptable for some salad dressings. Unrefined corn oil emits a wonderful fragrance for popping corn, but most American consumers find it too strong for their taste buds.

Buying olive oil comes with some additional caveats. Most olive oil sold in the United States is labeled either "extra-virgin" or "virgin," but it may be neither. Because Americans favor lighter-colored and less intensely flavored oils, much of the olive oil sold here is extra-virgin mixed

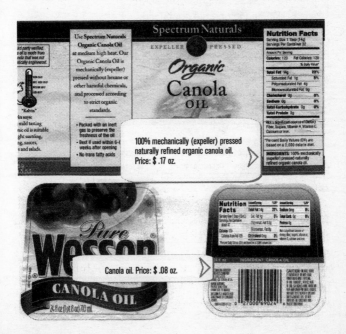

with virgin oil that has been refined and bleached. The best rule of thumb for buying olive oil is to purchase extra-virgin from a smaller company. This, of course, may not always be possible and is often expensive.

If your main motivation is truly healthy, wholesome eating, the organic label does not always serve as a reliable guide, but it *may* indicate fewer pesticide residues.

Shopping Tip

Health advocates make the following suggestions for buying any oil. Buy oil that has been:

- Processed at temperatures below 118°F
- Processed excluding light and air
- Processed without toxic solvents
- Bottled in opaque containers
- Bottled so that the air inside has been replaced by inert gas[8]

Best Bets

Beans, Nuts, Oil	Number of Current Pesticide Residues	Number of Environmental Contaminants	Availability of Organic		Price Comparison Per Pound January '05	
			National Brands*	Local**	Organic	Conventional
✓Kidney Beans	2	0	W	W	$1.59	$1.29
✓Split Peas	6	1	W	W	$1.19	$1.29
Mixed Nuts, no Peanuts***	16	12	L	L	$7.99+	$5.99
Dry Roasted Peanuts	20	9	W	W	$2.96	$3.00

Beans, Nuts, Oil	Number of Current Pesticide Residues	Number of Environmental Contaminants	Availability of Organic		Price Comparison Per Pound January '05	
			National Brands*	Local**	Organic	Conventional
Peanut Butter	23	12	W	W	$3.49	$2.59
Olive/Safflower Oil****	19	11	W	W	$ .17/oz.	$ .08/oz.

✓ = Best Bet for conventional

Source for Contaminants and Residues: FDA's Total Diet Study, 2002

* W = widely available; L = limited availability; H = hard to find; N/A = not available

** Seasonally available

*** Organic mixed nuts are unavailable. Individual organic nuts are available from $7.99 to $10.69 per pound.

**** The only way the Total Diet Study lists oil.

Bean, Nut, Seed, and Oil Production Comparison: Conventional versus Organic

		Conventional	Organic
Fertilizer Use	Beans	little synthetic nitrogen, moderate amounts of synthetic phosphorus, potassium	manures, compost, rock dust, cover cropping, crop rotation, green manuring
	Seeds	moderate amounts of synthetic phosphorus, nitrogen, and potassium	same as above
	Nuts	little need for fertilizer	little need for fertilizer

Bean, Nut, Seed, and Oil Production Comparison (Continued)

		Conventional	Organic
Pesticide Use	Beans	few synthetic insecticides, some use of fungicides, higher amount of herbicides	some use of organic pesticides, crop rotation
	Seeds	low amount of pesticide use	same as above
	Nuts	more pesticide use than for other crops, but half of all use is allowed for organic	much reliance on oil, some sulfur and copper use
Post-Harvest Handling	Edible Beans	little handling, except for processing peanut butter	little handling
	Edible Seeds	little handling	little handling
	Edible Nuts	little handling	little handling
	Oil Beans and Seeds	considerable amount of processing; numerous chemical additives	considerable amount of processing; few chemical additives

CONSUMER'S GUIDE

Aisle 3: Seeds, Beans, Nuts, and Oils

- Look for the USDA organic seal on all beans, nuts, and seeds.
- Seek out organic oils high in omega-3 fatty acids packed in opaque bottles.
- Avoid solvent-extracted oil.
- Avoid foods made with organic palm fruit oil.

- Buy beans, nuts, and seeds from bulk bins.
- Avoid nuts from distant farms (Brazil nuts, cashews, etc.).

- Seek out Fair Trade imported nuts.

- Seek out olive oil from small family farms making only first-pressed oil.

AVAILABILITY LEGEND

❶ Internet, Mail order **❷** Locally **Ⓡ** Regionally **❸** Statewide

AISLE 3 GUIDE TO BRANDS

Company Logo	Contact/Corporate Information	Company Logo	Contact/Corporate Information
	Amy's Kitchen Petaluma, CA 94953 707-578-7188 Independently owned amys.com		**Great Eastern Sun One World** Asheville, NC 28806 800-334-5809 great-eastern-sun.com
	Apollo Olive Oil Oregon House, CA 95962 530-692-2314 Family owned apollooliveoil.com ❶		**Hearty & Natural** Hope, MN 56046 800-297-5997 Sunrich Stake Technologies sunrich.com
	**Bionaturae** North Franklin, CT 06254 860-642-6996 Family owned bionaturae.com		**I. M. Healthy** Glenview, IL 60025 800-288-1012 Soy Nut Butter Company soynutbutter.com
	Dawes Hill Honey 888-800-8075 Once Again Nut Butter onceagainnutbutter.com		**Island Organics** Honoka'a, HI 96727 808-775-8115 Family owned islandorganics.com
	Eden Foods Clinton, MI 49236 888-424-EDEN Independently owned eden-foods.com	Living Tree Community	**Living Tree Community Foods** Berkley, CA 94709 510-526-7106 livingtreecommunity.com
FRONTIER 	**Frontier Natural Products Co-op** Norway, IA 52318 800-729-5422 Farmer co-op frontiercoop.com		**Long Meadow Ranch** St. Helena, CA 94574 707-963-4555 longmeadowranch.com
	Futters Nut Butters Buffalo Grove, IL 60089 847-634-6976 futtersnutbutters.com ❶		**Loriva** San Leandro, CA 94577 510-686-0116 Nspired Natural Foods nspiredfoods.com
	Gaeta 800-669-2681 Gaeta Imports gaetaimports.com		**Native Forest** Carpinteria, CA 93014 805-684-8500 Edward & Sons Trading Co. edwardandsons.com

AISLE 3 GUIDE TO BRANDS

Company Logo	Contact/Corporate Information	Company Logo	Contact/Corporate Information
	Nature's Approved Hartsdale, NY 10530 914-428-6800 Assured Organics assuredorganics.com		**Spectrum Organic Products, Inc.** Petaluma, CA 94954 800-995-2705 spectrumorganics.com
	Olio Beato Scarsdale, NY 10583 914-723-5850 Pietro DeMarco Importers organicoil.com		**Sun West Organics** Davis, CA 95616 530-758-8550 sunwestfoods.com
	Rigoni Organic Oxford, CT 06478 203-267-3280 Rigoni USA rigoniusa.com		**Sunstone Vineyards** Santa Ynez, CA 93460 805-688-9463 Family owned sunstonewinery.com
	Santa Barbara Olive Co. Santa Barbara, CA 93117 800-624-4896 Family owned sbolive.com 		**Supremo Oil** Hayward, CA 94545 510-732-8072 supremooil.com
	Seapoint Farms Huntington Beach, CA 92648 714-841-9831 seapointfarms.com		**Tehama Gold** Flournoy, CA 96029 530-833-0119 Homegrown Enterprises tehamagold.com
	ShariAnn's Organic Garden City, NY 11530 800-434-4246 Hain-Celestial Heinz shariannsorganic.com		**Westbrae Natural** Garden City, NY 11530 800-434-4246 Hain-Celestial Heinz westbrae.com

AISLE 4
The Dairy Case

OF ALL THE FOODS we eat today, dairy tops the list for appealing to food faddists. Some urge consumers to avoid dairy products altogether; others lobby for raw, unpasteurized milk. While the familiar "Got Milk?" promotion trumpets its benefits,[1] organic advocates hammer away at conventional milk's deficiencies. Somewhere amid the clamor and conviction lies the truth.

The fact is that most Americans do get milk, ignoring the warnings of antidairy activists: in 2001 we produced 169.7 billion pounds of dairy goods.[2] As one of the faster-growing segments of the organic industry, dairy benefits greatly from all the attention given to cows and their products, achieving 58 percent annual sales increases.[3]

With all the bad press the dairy business gets, one detail remains underreported: dairy farmers care about cows. Anyone who chooses to spend sixteen hours a day, 363 days a year with members of the bovine persuasion has to love 'em. The remaining two days? Many farmers spend their "vacations" at the county fair showing off their prized animals and casting envious eyes at the winners. When critics hurl pernicious charges at the "dairy industry," it is important to remember that most dairy farmers work extremely hard in a very competitive market. To blame them for the problems related to the industry as a whole is both disingenuous and inaccurate. From the consumer's standpoint, however, some of these charges warrant attention.

There are six major issues concerning the dairy industry:

- Pesticide residues
- Drug residues
- Injected growth hormones
- Animal welfare
- Manure management
- Pathogenic microorganisms

PESTICIDE RESIDUES

For years the organic movement has complained about the presence of chemical residues in milk. The theory is that cows eat conventionally grown feed, and pesticides end up in the milk they produce. There are four basic forms of feed: corn and soybeans, hay, silage, and pasture. Pastures and hay usually don't get sprayed, and most corn grain is somewhat protected by its husks. On the other hand, corn silage might harbor pesticides because it is made from exposed parts of the plant—stalks, leaves, husks, and ears.

Once in an animal's body, pesticide residues migrate into fat cells, so whole milk, cream, and butter provide a residue-rich environment. But the U.S. milk supply contains very few residues from currently used pesticides. The USDA's Pesticide Data Program tested for sixty-nine different pesticides or their metabolites (breakdown products). Out of 595 whole-milk samples collected from nine states, the PDP found eighty-nine residues. Eighty-two of the eighty-nine were metabolites of the long-banned DDT[4]—a persistent pesticide that contaminates parts of the food chain in very small amounts.

Of the remaining seven residues found in milk, six of them are not listed in the Code of Federal Regulations, which means the EPA finds the residue safe enough not to have a tolerance listing. All of the residue levels, including the DDT metabolite, were well below the EPA tolerance levels. There is no evidence that today's organic practices protect food from environmental contaminants. Organic milk is just as susceptible to the ghosts of DDT and present-day air pollution as is conventional milk.

DRUG RESIDUES

Antibiotics are given to cows to treat mastitis—an infection of the udder—and any discussion about organic milk soon turns to this topic. Organic promoters frequently imply that conventional milk contains antibiotics. For example, in *The Food Revolution,* John Robbins writes, "Antibiotics allowed in U.S. cow's milk: 80."[5] This is simply not true. What he probably meant was "Number of commercial brands of antibiotics approved for use in cows: 80." It's true that antibiotics top the list of bovine medications, but here we must make the distinction between drugs given to cows and what actually shows up in the milk we drink.

So how is it that farmers can give their cows large doses of drugs and then not have them show up in milk? What goes in must come out, right? Are regulators participating in some grand cover-up? The answer is that drugs do show up in milk, but cows' milk is one of the most regulated commodities sold in the United States. Antibiotic residues are not tolerated, and milk that is found to contain them is diverted to a septic waste system and never sold (see sidebar on next page). Because they lose money every time milk goes down the drain, dairy farmers exercise extreme caution when administering antibiotics and are often reluctant to use them.

Antibiotic abuse in agriculture—and its role in creating resistant strains of bacteria—represents a cause for genuine concern, but if you are solely driven by worries about antibiotic residues *in milk,* you are the victim of a kind of fear-mongering found on numerous websites.

TESTING FOR ANTIBIOTICS

It's a fact—dairies can't sell milk that contains even minute traces of antibiotics.

When it comes to antibiotic residues in milk, do dairy processing plants trust that all farmers do the right thing? No. Because one truck may hold milk from several farms, milk from each farm's bulk tanks is sampled before loading. The milk from the truck is then tested at the bottling plant before being pumped into storage tanks. This is done not only to protect consumers, but because even a small amount of antibiotics (less than one part per billion) kills the good bacteria used to make other dairy products such as cheese, butter, and yogurt.

If detectable antibiotic residues show up in the truck's tank, the entire load is dumped and each farmer's sample is then tested to find the offender. The farmer responsible for the contamination must pay for the entire load. Usually the next time the farmer contaminates a load, the production facility refuses to buy from him again.[6] Given the price fluctuation in the industry, dairies of any size cannot afford to have residues show up in their milk. This isn't just about being nice to consumers or following the law; it's about being able to pay the light bill.[7]

HORMONES

Recombinant bovine growth hormone (rBGH) jumped into the headlines in 1993 when the FDA approved Monsanto's Posilac. The use of this hormone is often portrayed as something new, but farmers have been using BST (the naturally occurring form) since the 1940s, when it was extracted—in a slow and expensive process—from the pituitary glands of slaughtered cattle. Today's hormone is not extracted; rather, it is the much more efficient product of biotechnology.

MORE THAN rBST

Genetically engineered bovine somatotropin is not the only hormone given to cows in conventional dairies. Prostaglandin F2d induces cows to go into heat (for impregnation); gonadotropin treats cystic ovarian disease in higher producing cows; and oxytocin stimulates the cow to release her milk (milk letdown). Oxytocin is the only hormone allowed in organic production. These hormones presumably have the same potential as rBST for winding up in our milk, but critics haven't paid much attention to them.

You see this hormone listed several different ways. The bovine growth hormone that a cow secretes is called bovine somatotropin. (Humans secrete human somatotropin.) BST or BGH refers to the natural hormone. The addition of the lowercase r (as in rBST or rBGH) indicates the genetically engineered (recombinant) hormone.

All cows produce bovine somatotropin (BST), just not in the exaggerated amounts given to them with rBST. Although it allows cows to produce 10 to 15 percent more milk, critics charge—and Monsanto (the manufacturer of Posilac) admits—that cows injected with rBST have increased health problems such as mastitis, which leads to more antibiotic use.[8]

In addition to the potential health problems, treated cows have a slightly lower life expectancy (three to four years). It's true that an organic cow may live and produce a little longer, but in both organic and conventional cows, yields drop after the first few productive years. The reason conventional cows produce for only three or four years is that farmers, many of whom are struggling with tight profit margins, cannot afford to keep a low-yielding cow. Old Bossie that gave you milk for breakfast is destined to become

hamburger for your dinner. Farmers call it culling, and organic farmers cull their cows, too.

Although consumers may be somewhat concerned about
the effects of rBST on cows, we are more troubled by what
it might do to us. As happens with many new products,
critics immediately produced a litany of potential health
problems. Studies have linked rBST with a decrease in milk's
protein and an increase in its fat content. Some critics have
also charged rBST with contributing to diabetes, obesity,
and hypertension. Others see it as much ado about nothing.
Julie Miller-Jones, a professor of Nutrition and Food Safety
at the College of St. Catherine in St. Paul, Minnesota,
puts it bluntly: "It is not cost effective to buy higher priced
organic or specialty milk, because there is no effect on the
nutritional quality or the safety of milk from cows treated
with rBGH or antibiotics."[9]

Not every farmer uses rBST. A survey conducted by the
USDA's National Health Monitoring System found that
dairy farms with more than five hundred cows are most
likely to use hormones. Issued in 2002, the report stated:
"Nationally, 15.2 percent of the herds were using rBST at
the time of the Dairy 2002 study while 22.3 percent of
cows received the hormone. Although the increase in rBST
use was observed in all herd sizes, cows in large herds were
given the hormone 6.2 times more often than those in
small herds. The use of rBST was greater in the Western
region than in the other regions."[10]

In small dairies with less than a hundred cows, only
8.8 percent used the hormone.[11] In some states, small
dairies constitute 80 percent or more of all dairies. Critics
create the impression that large dairies routinely inject
rBST into all the cows in a herd. This is false. Farmers use
rBST on an "as needed" basis in cows with falling production. Only certain cows in a herd will be given rBST at any
one time.

THE STORY OF BST AND IGF-1

All mammals produce growth hormones (in cows, BST) that are processed by the liver into insulinlike growth factor (IGF-1). This is a good thing. It helps the body grow and regenerate cells. But critics of the dairy industry charge that giving additional growth hormones to cows increases the amount of IGF-1 in humans when dairy products are consumed. This, they say, is a bad thing. Since IGF-1 was first isolated in the 1950s as a potential treatment for dwarfism, thousands of studies have been conducted on IGF-1 and rBST. The results seem to depend on who is paying for the studies.

The problem with IGF-1 derived from the growth hormones of cows is that it didn't work in humans, whether injected or taken orally (important when considering the criticisms of rBST in milk).[12] Although studies with rats showed some effect—even if taken orally—there is no conclusive proof about its effect on humans[13]—which leads to the current controversy about whether you should be taking IGF-1 or avoiding it. Dr. Samuel Epstein, for instance, insists that IGF-1 increases the risk of breast, prostate, and colon cancer, citing a correlation between high levels of IGF-1 and these particular cancers.[14] Despite claims (and studies) such as these, websites and health food stores actively sell IGF-1 touting its ability to reverse aging, build muscles, and prevent cancer. They also cite studies to prove their claims.

FDA rBST Guidelines for Milk Product Labels

In the store, you may be able to find labels that identify milk from untreated cows. Despite lobbying from the dairy industry and Monsanto, some bottling plants have found it profitable to label such milk. Here is an example:

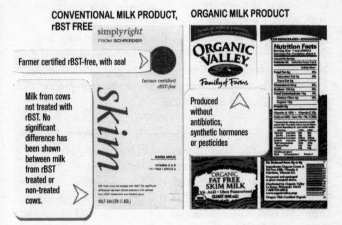

The FDA has issued guidelines regarding these claims: "food manufacturers who do not use milk from cows treated with recombinant bovine somatotropin (rBST) may voluntarily inform consumers of this fact on their product labels or labeling, *provided that the statements are truthful and not misleading*" (emphasis added). The FDA insists that:

- The following statement must appear on the label of both organic milk and milk produced without rBST: "The Federal government has determined that rBST/rBGH milk is safe for humans and cows, and that no significant difference has been shown between milk from rBST/rBGH treated or non rBST/rBGH treated cows."

- "No hormones" and "hormone free" are false claims because all milk contains naturally occurring hormones, and milk cannot be processed in a manner that renders it free of hormones. "No added hormones" is also misleading because rBST is not added to the milk, it is given to the cow.
- A milk label cannot say "no antibiotics," "no antibiotics added," or "antibiotic free" because *no milk* can legally contain antibiotics.
- An organic milk label should not say "produced without pesticides" or simply "no pesticides" because organic milk producers use *approved* pesticides.
- The FDA does not recognize any certification program other than the USDA's NOP.

All this said, rBST's days may be numbered. By early 2004, Monsanto had run into difficulties maintaining a sterile environment at its Austrian production facility, so it cut production and rationed rBST among dairy farmers. Monsanto has indicated that full production may not resume anytime soon, although it had increased somewhat by December 2004.

Some observers suggested that Monsanto was attempting to wean dairy farmers from overusing rBST.[15] Other dairy industry commentators speculate that the reduction in rBST was responsible for the dramatic increase in milk prices that consumers experienced during the spring and summer of 2004. Although an interesting theory, the increase in prices is more likely the result of producers' efforts to reduce the milk supply.[16]

ANIMAL WELFARE

Animal welfare involves the drugs cows are given, the feed they eat, and the homes they live in. In most cases, an individual animal's comfort relates directly to the number of cows on the farm. Organic dairy operations, with a few exceptions, have small herds, allowing farmers more time to pamper each cow. This pampering frequently takes the form of rotational grazing in well-maintained green grass pastures. Adequate barn space makes for healthier cows, although NOP regulations do not specify space requirements. Most conventional dairy farms also maintain small herds and treat their animals well. Every dairy farmer, whether organic or conventional, faces tough competition, and most farmers with small operations cannot afford to mistreat their cows.

In factorylike dairies with more than five hundred cows, problems—such as cramped spaces with no access to pastures, use of antibiotics to keep cows healthy, and hormones to keep them productive—are the rule, not the exception. This environment is not conducive to contented cows. It is a fact: happy, healthy, stress-free cows produce more milk.

MANURE MANAGEMENT

The average milking cow produces eighty pounds of manure every day, *plus* contaminated bedding. While all livestock farmers must manage manure, the clean environment required for milking means dairy farmers have to deal with it daily. For them, manure simply cannot be ignored. In the past, farm boys armed with a pitchfork and shovel pitched the manure and straw bedding into a heap behind the barn and spread it on the fields in the spring.

By the 1940s, most new dairy barns built a trough in the floor directly behind the standing cow. This trough ran the length of the barn and contained a conveyer belt that carried the manure out of the barn and dumped it onto a growing pile. Most small dairies and nearly all organic dairies still use this system. The larger megadairies now use a flushing system that sends manure and a lot of added water to a holding lagoon, which is pumped out several times a year for use as fertilizer.

Presently, there are only a handful of very large organic dairies; the average has fewer than ninety cows. Most of these dairies have extensive grazing pastures where wastes are naturally deposited on the land. Whatever is collected from the milking barn is incorporated into the farm's overall soil management plan.

PATHOGENIC MICROORGANISMS

Of all the potential health problems related to dairy products, pathogens should be your biggest concern. Milk provides a perfect place for bacteria to grow, and contamination at the farm happens in a number of ways. For example, it doesn't take much of an anatomical imagination to realize that milk and manure originate in roughly the same place. Contaminated udders constitute the largest source of bacteria in milk, followed by infected human handlers.[17] Organic milk is just as susceptible to this type of contamination as conventional milk. Pasteurization (allowed under the NOP rule) kills these critters, which is the reason why raw (unpasteurized) milk can be dangerous.

Although they are not technically pathogens, a related problem involves something called somatic cells, which are measured by the somatic cell count (SCC). These fleshy cells from inside the teat are sloughed off during milking and may be accompanied by an elevated white blood cell count. The problem with a high cell count in milk is that it decreases the protein level, which leads to lower-quality dairy products. Dairy farmers often refer to milk with a high SCC as "dirty milk." When an SCC gets too high (300,000 or more), conventional dairies administer antibiotics. If they cannot control a high SCC, the cow is usually culled from the herd. If many of the cows in the herd produce a high SCC, then the milk is not allowed in fluid milk products (although it is allowed in manufactured products such as powdered milk).

To combat a high SCC, organic dairies use several natural remedies. NOP standards require a cow with a count of more than 400,000 to be culled from the herd. Culled organic cows are either sold to conventional dairies or slaughtered for organic beef. Several studies have linked organic milk with higher SCCs than conventional milk.[18]

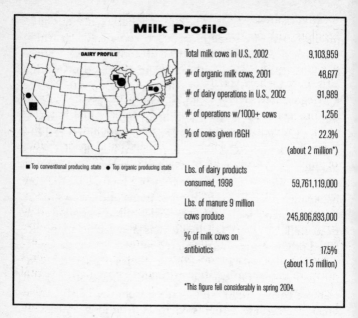

Milk Profile

Total milk cows in U.S., 2002	9,103,959
# of organic milk cows, 2001	48,677
# of dairy operations in U.S., 2002	91,989
# of operations w/1000+ cows	1,256
% of cows given rBGH	22.3%
	(about 2 million*)
Lbs. of dairy products consumed, 1998	59,761,119,000
Lbs. of manure 9 million cows produce	245,806,893,000
% of milk cows on antibiotics	17.5%
	(about 1.5 million)

DAIRY PROFILE

■ Top conventional producing state   ● Top organic producing state

*This figure fell considerably in spring 2004.

Size Matters

Although there is a lot of debate about the effects of pesticides, antibiotics, and hormones, one thing remains clear: many of the problems can be alleviated with smaller farms. Although new technologies and equipment have allowed dairy farmers to increase herd sizes, there is a point at which the family dairy ceases to be a farm and turns into a factory.

The good news, despite what critics say, is that the majority of American dairy farms remain small family operations. In 2002 the USDA listed 91,989 dairy farms operating in the United States with an average of ninety-nine cows each.[19] In general, large population centers depend on huge herds. California, with 35 million people, has the largest dairy factories. These operations confine their cows to feedlots with no access to green pastures. Each dairy may have two thousand to five thousand cows. If you want to see cow abuse, manure pollution, and out-of-control mastitis, here's where you'll find it.

Regrettably, factory-sized organic dairies do exist, drawing fire from traditional organic advocates. Mark Kastel of the Cornucopia Institute of Wisconsin, took aim by filing a federal lawsuit in January 2005 against Aurora Dairies of Platteville, Colorado. Kastel charged that Aurora, with over 5,000 cows, used the NOP loophole on access to outdoors (see Aisle 5) to confine their cows to dry feedlots. Aurora claims access to pasture would degrade the land in Colorado's arid high plains. But less than twenty-five miles away from Platteville, veterinarians Meg Cattell and Arden Nelson's 400 cows on one thousand certified acres seem to get along just fine without major environmental degradation.

A flurry of news stories about Aurora's feedlots appeared, but most media outlets ignored one of the more egregious aspects of Aurora's process. Aurora Organic Dairy's milk is not destined for their own milk cartons, but rather for cartons featuring private labels. The result: Costco now features organic milk in ultra-pasteurized six gallon packs with a "sell-by" window of more than six weeks. Many organic advocates cannot believe six-week-old milk still qualifies as organic.

BUYING MILK

With more than ninety thousand dairies of various sizes in the United States, it seems unfair to make blanket statements about all dairies based on the problems associated with large dairy factories. Although large farms confine cows and rely on antibiotics and growth hormones, these operations comprise only 3 percent of the dairy industry, and smaller dairies are still the norm.

The West is one region of the country that will continue to expand the size of its herds. For example, milk produced in the southern California basin is more likely to be managed with rBST and no green grass.[20] Other states with similar large herds include Arizona, Florida, Idaho, New Mexico, and Washington. If you live in these states, consider buying organic milk.

Shopping Tip

When buying fresh fluid milk, the size of the herd may be more important than whether it is organic or conventional. Smaller farms have more time to care for cows, cull for mastitis, restrict drug and hormone use, and deal with waste in an ecologically sound manner. Of course, most organic dairy farms fall into this category, but large-scale organic dairy farms do exist. Your own organic priorities (i.e., health risks, environmental impact, animal welfare) and where you live may help you determine if milk is where you want to spend your organic food dollar.

States in other regions of the country have low average herd sizes of one hundred cows or less. To put it in perspective, Wisconsin has more than 19,000 dairies, whereas California has only 2,500. These smaller farms are less likely to use hormones and antibiotics. Also, smaller herds have less impact on the environment. It is a safe bet that Milwaukee, Madison, Minneapolis, and Chicago all have abundant supplies of conventional milk from small herds. The same would be true for many eastern population centers.

A growing number of organic dairy farmers now offer raw milk, because raw milk advocates claim that pasteurization destroys enzymes, vitamins, proteins, and friendly bacteria. Possibly. But pasteurization also kills deadly microorganisms, which are by far the greatest threat to your health among the major dairy issues.

If you are still concerned about the safety of conventional milk, *Consumer Reports* expressed it well in January 2000:

> There are many reasons consumers may choose to buy organic milk. But should they fear serving regular milk to their kids? No ... Organic milk may also be for you if you want to support organic farming principles. But we see no reason to buy it for fear that regular milk is unsafe to drink.[21]

Goat Milk

One way to avoid the cow milk controversy is to drink goat milk. As far as your health is concerned, goat milk's smaller fat globules digest more easily, and the milk contains more calcium with fewer saturated fats.

In other respects, goats aren't much different from cows and are subject to the same problems with bacteria. The same holds true for somatic cells. In fact, the SCC standard for goat milk is twice what it is for cows (800,000). Whereas 93 percent of cow herds meet the standards, 50 to

65 percent of the goat herds fail.[22] Despite this fact, as much as 70 percent of the world's population consumes goat milk and cheese.

Buying Goat Milk

Although there are approximately 1.5 million goats in the United States, goat milk can be difficult to find. In large metropolitan areas, nonorganic goat milk may be available in natural food stores and some supermarkets, but organic is rarely available. Consumers interested in organic goat products may be able to buy directly from a farm.

BUTTER

Nothing beats the taste of real butter, but its high saturated fat content leads many consumers to just say no. Although Americans have cut their consumption of butter by 20 percent over the last thirty years, we still managed to eat more than a billion pounds of it in 1997.[23]

As if clogging your arteries weren't enough to worry about, critics claim that butterfat is a storehouse for pesticides. Since certain toxins tend to migrate to fat cells (they are lipophilic, or "fat loving"), butter—which is at least 85 percent fat—provides the perfect place for pesticides to hide.

Testing reveals that conventional butter contains more than just currently used pesticides. The FDA's 2003 Total Diet Study found thirty different chemical contaminants in conventional butter:

Type of Contaminant	Number of Chemicals Found	Percentage with Residues	Total Number of Residues Found
Currently registered pesticides	7	21%	53
Banned pesticides	8	32%	131
Nonpesticidal chemicals	15	47%	181
Total chemicals found	30		

Advocates suggest that organic production methods have a positive impact on what residues show up in an animal's fat. Maybe. Let's consider what's in butter.

Organic milk producers feed their cows certified organic feed. No prohibited pesticides are allowed, either in the growing, preparation, or storage of the cows' food. Nearly all conventional medications are prohibited, and the barn's pest control measures are closely monitored. This then would seem to limit the amount of contamination found in organic butter.

But what holds true for organic butter holds true for all organic foods: they may be lower in residues from currently used pesticides, but they are not free from old pesticides or a polluted environment.

One such environmental contaminant is PCBs. PCBs were used in products such as fluorescent lights, electrical devices, microscopes, and hydraulic oils. PCBs are linked to cancer and dysfunction of the immune, reproductive, nervous, and endocrine systems. Banned in 1977, residues still routinely show up. Although the amounts are declining, in 2002 Health Canada reported finding 264 parts per trillion in butter samples. In fact, butter is second only to fish in harboring PCBs.

Buying Butter

Feed is the key to what kind of butter (or milk) you might consider buying. The more green pasture a cow is allowed to eat, the more conjugated linoleic acid (CLA) its milk products will contain. CLA is a naturally occurring fatty acid component of beef, milk, and other foods. Derived from linolenic acid, it is an essential omega-6 fatty acid. Several research studies suggest that CLA helps prevent cancers, reduces plaque formation in the blood, and possibly enhances the human immune system.

Because the dairy industry has shifted to a grain-based diet, the amount of this kind of CLA in our diets has fallen considerably over the last twenty years. Dairy researchers have documented that the percentage of CLA in the milk fat derived from fresh pastured cows is more than double that of cows fed a grain-based diet. The more grain fed to cows, the greater the milk production but the lower the CLA content.[24]

Organic rules require that cows have access to the outdoors, and many certifiers require maintained pastures, but neither restricts grain as feed nor requires fresh grass. Organic methods cannot guarantee grass-fed cows exclusively, so if you are concerned about CLA, look for butter made from the milk of grass-fed cows, organic or not.

THE POWER OF CHEESE

Americans really like cheese. In February 2003 alone we consumed almost 655 million pounds of it.[25] Sales of organic cheese are rising at unusually high rates for the food industry, and most organic dairies have trouble meeting the demand. Making organic cheese isn't easy because the technology has radically changed during the last decade.

Although organic milk is available, the problem lies in obtaining the other ingredients.

Of the three basic ingredients that go into making cheese, milk constitutes 99.99 percent.[26] So if you have organic milk, making organic cheese should be easy. All you have to do is add salt, cultures, and rennet—an enzyme used for thousands of years to cause the protein in milk to coagulate, form curds, and separate from the whey (the watery part of milk). And that's the problem. In the last twenty years, the cheese industry has phased out its use of natural rennet and now relies on recombinant Chymosin, a genetically engineered substance. About 70 percent of all cheese in the United States is made with recombinant Chymosin.[27] Organic rules prohibit the use of *any* GEOs.

Finding GEO-free rennet is difficult, so organic cheese producers must request letters of confirmation from their suppliers that the enzymes and cultures are GEO free. These letters are often cloaked in vaguely worded phrasing to absolve suppliers and producers of any legal responsibility.

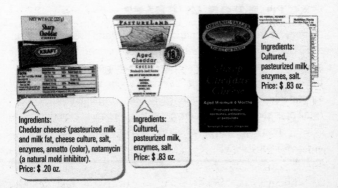

Ingredients:
Cheddar cheeses (pasteurized milk and milk fat, cheese culture, salt, enzymes, annatto (color), natamycin (a natural mold inhibitor).
Price: $ .20 oz.

Ingredients:
Cultured, pasteurized milk, enzymes, salt.
Price: $ .83 oz.

Ingredients:
Cultured, pasteurized milk, enzymes, salt.
Price: $ .83 oz.

Taste Check: Cheese

We sampled three different sharp cheddar cheeses: one conventional, one grass fed, and one organic. For taste and "meltability," the grass-fed, locally produced cheese won the day hands down, but the organic held its own. Comparisons to the conventional cheese almost seemed unfair. As with peanut butter and finely crafted bread, the products really resemble each other in name only.

Buying Cheese

Cheese is subject to the same assaults as milk, with additional concerns about Chymosin. The only way to avoid GEOs or *added* hormones is to buy organic cheese. If organic is unavailable, then high-quality, locally produced artisan cheese—because much of it is produced by small-herd dairies—provides a tasty, environmentally sound alternative.

BACTINE FOR CHEESE?

Natamycin (also called Pimaricin) is a food additive similar to an antibiotic that many conventional producers used to prevent mold from growing on the surface of packaged cheeses. After the cheese is cut to the final size, the pieces are sprayed with or dipped into a solution of natamycin. Some organically certified retail operations allow natamycin in the wax layer covering artisan cheeses, but it is not on the NOP's National List of approved substances.

Nearly 90 percent of all milk produced on Wisconsin's comparatively small dairy farms is made into cheese,[28] so any cheese from Wisconsin is a good bet. (It also leads the nation in organic dairies.) New York, Minnesota, Pennsylvania, and other states tend to have smaller herds as well.

Many of the national brands of conventional cheese are made in California, which manufactured 1.06 billion pounds of cheese in 2001.[29] Unfortunately, most of the milk there comes from large dairy operations. When these monster dairy herds overproduce, the milk ends up in cheese, powdered milk, and canned condensed milk. It might take a bit more work and time on your part, but reading the label on your cheese may reveal its milk source.

YOGURT

Human beings have been eating yogurt since about 2000 B.C.E., but it wasn't until 1970 that yogurt began its life as a mainstream health food in the United States. Stories abound about people in Bulgaria, Turkey, and Tibet practically living forever on yogurt because of the "friendly" bacteria it contains. These tales have not been lost on the dairy industry, which has since promoted yogurt as a "probiotic."

To meet the legal definition of yogurt, it must contain at least two bacteria, *Lactobacillus bulgaricus* and *Streptococcus thermophilus*—although other strains (*Streptococcus lactis, S. cremoris, Lactobacillus acidophilus,* and *L. plantarum*) can also be used. These bacteria form yogurt's distinctive flavor and custardlike texture. Because we need *L. acidophilus* in our gastrointestinal tracts, yogurt producers highlight its presence, but they rarely list *S. lactis.*

Buying Yogurt

A number of national and regional brands offer organic yogurt and should be easy to find in all co-ops and natural food chains, and most supermarkets. As with all finished dairy products, yogurt is only as good as the milk it starts with, so pay close attention to brands—especially regional or local—that make use of milk from smaller herds.

If you eat yogurt to populate your intestines with good bacteria, note the cultures listed on the label. And while you're at it, you may want to check for excessive amounts of sugar. If you like sweet, fruity yogurt, you will save money and have a healthier product by buying plain yogurt and adding your own fruit.

If it's delicious, fatty calories you want (to avoid), look (out) for several organic brands now offering whole milk, cream-on-the-top varieties. They're tasty, sure, but—you know where this is going.

ICE CREAM

According to existing USDA regulation, ice cream must have at least 10 percent butterfat. It can also have 9 percent milk solids, 12 percent sweeteners, 55 percent water, and no more than 0.5 percent stabilizers and emulsifiers. Consumers might think the milk solids are from fresh milk, but they are usually from concentrated skimmed milk or powder. Recently the industry has substituted blends of whey protein concentrates, caseinates, and whey powders.

Organic ice cream was once hard to find, but by 2004 most of the national organic dairies—Alta Dena, Ben & Jerry's, Cascadian Farms, Julie's Organic Ice Cream, Cascade Glacier Ice Cream, and Stonyfield Farm—had added it to their product mix. A better bet would be to seek out small, local organic dairies such as Sibby's Premium in the upper Midwest, Straus Family Creamery on the West Coast, or Bart's Homemade in Massachusetts.

SOY DAIRY PRODUCTS

Soymilk originated in China and Japan, where real dairy products were unknown until the last fifty years. William Shurtleff and Akiko Aoyagi, in *The Book of Tofu,* describe the incredibly widespread cottage industry that soy became in Japan, permeating the entire culture.[30] Until recently, every neighborhood had its own shop selling fresh warm soymilk and tofu. This Japanese staple has become a worldwide phenomenon. The hundreds of products made from soybeans now far surpass the number of animal dairy products available.

Organic soymilk has enjoyed tremendous success in the last decade. A plethora of brands now grace the dairy case and grocery shelves in aseptic cartons with extended shelf life. Despite all the branding, over 40 percent of the soymilk for sale in the United States originates from just one plant in southern Minnesota. Here's how it's made.

A Hilum of Beans

Soybean varieties are defined by a little piece of plant anatomy called the hilum, which attaches a bean or pea to its pod. In most legumes, the hilum simply falls off when the bean dries and is of no further consequence. But in some soybean varieties, this little part has different colors: clear, yellow, gray, buff, brown, or black. The color of the hilum indicates the quality of the bean. Soy products like milk and tofu are made from the clear or yellow bean varieties, also known as "food-grade" soybeans.

Until the late 1990s, food-grade varieties accounted for less than 10 percent of all soybean production in the United States. But demand for soy products—especially milk—has raised this number to more than 15 percent of the market. While conventional feed-grade beans often bring around $4.50 per bushel, organic food-grade beans hover at $20.00 a bushel—a strong incentive for conventional farmers to go organic.

However, only high-quality, "identity preserved" (non-GEO) beans fetch this premium price, and it takes most new organic farmers several years to get the hang of growing top-quality organic beans. Most farmers must be content with twelve to fifteen dollars per bushel for the first several years.

Making Soymilk

The first step in making soymilk is removing the seed coat or hull, which can produce bitter, yellow milk. To remove the hull, whole beans are soaked in water, then ground into a smooth paste. The finer the grind, the smoother the milk. Many processors then cook the milk to get rid of the beany flavor. As with any heating process, some nutrient loss occurs.

The pasty slurry is then filtered, pressed, and centrifuged. In the past, soymilk was bottled at this point with no further processing. The Japanese still prefer soymilk in this form, but American consumers tend to like the mouthfeel they associate with dairy products, so U.S. soymilk processors often add vegetable oil, sweeteners, and salt for creaminess and taste.

Soymilk's nutrients are similar to those of animal milk,

providing about the same fat, calories, and protein. Soymilk also contains estrogenic hormones, which critics have suggested might disrupt the body's normal hormone levels, citing higher rates of asthma, allergies, thyroid disorders, calcium deficiencies, and reproductive disorders in people who drank soy-based formulas when they were babies.[31] This might be an important risk because 750,000 infants are fed soy-based formulas every year.

Despite critics' warnings, the soy formula industry insists that the long-term health outcomes are the same as for those infants consuming cow or human milk. On the other hand, other health activists cite these hormones as protection from breast cancer. In any case, the antisoy campaign has yet to gain traction with the general public, and American consumers now eat and drink hundreds of products made with soybeans and soymilk.

Buying Soymilk

For many years, the only place you could buy any kind of soymilk was in plastic bottles at Asian markets. Then it migrated to health and natural food stores in shelf-stable packages that can be stored unopened for months without refrigeration. Today supermarkets stock cartons of plain or flavored organic and conventional soymilk right next to cow's milk in the dairy case.

Is there any reason to reach for an organic-labeled soymilk instead of the cheaper conventional model? Healthwise, few pesticide residues lurk in soybeans. When testing for forty-three different pesticides in soybeans, the USDA found eleven. The three most frequently found were chlorpyrifos, dieldrin, and malathion. Forty-one percent of all 590 samples were contaminated with malathion. Research indicates that malathion moves rapidly out of the body by way of urine, feces, and expired air; it is not considered carcinogenic.[32] But forty-four samples contained the banned pesticide dieldrin, which is much more worrisome as a residue. Although not directly related to consumers' health, conventional soybean farmers use herbicides that can lead to groundwater contamination.

Another concern about conventional soybeans is the prevalence of genetically engineered varieties. By 2004, 85 percent of all soybeans planted in the United States were engineered. If you are worried about these varieties, organic beans offer assurance against consuming genetically engineered products.

Other dairy alternatives and soy products you'll find include tofu, tempeh, soy cheese, miso, soy yogurt, rice milk, almond milk, and oat milk.

THE CHICKEN OR THE EGG

For over five thousand years both chickens and eggs have been on our menus. The red jungle fowl, mother of all chicken breeds, still roams the rain forests of Malaysia. Its descendant, the chicken, is now the most commonly found domesticated animal in the world. Despite the genetic connection, the scrawny-looking bird wandering in the jungle bears little resemblance to the commercially bred laying hen or broiler.

Before the 1950s, chickens had the run of the whole farmyard, together with the dogs, cats, and kids, and their care was often left to women and children. This homey way of producing eggs is long gone. Today's conventional egg factories don't even have a farmyard, and the closest most children get to a laying hen is the carton in the refrigerator.

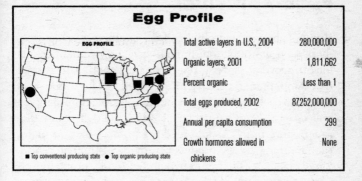

Egg Profile

Total active layers in U.S., 2004	280,000,000
Organic layers, 2001	1,811,662
Percent organic	Less than 1
Total eggs produced, 2002	87,252,000,000
Annual per capita consumption	299
Growth hormones allowed in chickens	None

■ Top conventional producing state ● Top organic producing state

Despite this lack of human-chicken interaction, Americans consumed about 87 billion eggs in 2002.[33] How does the egg industry produce this staggering figure? Massive flocks of layers—75,000 birds or more—make up 95 percent of U.S. egg production, and eight companies have flocks greater than five million birds.[34] The egg industry has frequently been criticized for how it supplies those billions of eggs. Critics cite the following issues:

- Feed additives
- Animal welfare

GET CRACKING

Eggs aren't just for breakfast anymore. "Shell eggs" (basically, large vats of cracked eggs) are used extensively in processed foods. To get these eggs, commercial producers use machines that process up to 65,000 eggs an hour. Shell fragments are filtered out, salt or sugar may be added, and all are required to be pasteurized. As organic production increases, so will the amount of organic shell eggs, produced in exactly the same manner.

FEED ADDITIVES

Rumors abound that chicken feed contains stimulants to increase egg production. In fact, drug enforcement agents have uncovered several operations attempting to extract methamphetamine from chicken feed.[35] This rumor can be put to roost: the FDA has never approved stimulants in chicken feed, and no one has succeeded in extracting much more from chicken feed than bran flakes. Actually, the last thing an egg producer wants is a stimulated bird. Chickens are easily frightened and naturally prone to hysteria. Hyper chickens lay fewer eggs and can sometimes stampede themselves into the corner of their cage and suffocate.

In order to lay eggs, chickens must have protein. Too little or too much—producers aim for around 25 percent—and the hen stops making eggs. Commercial feed contains grains of moderate protein content such as corn, barley, oats, or wheat, so it must be supplemented with higher-protein sources like alfalfa, soybeans, or the much-maligned animal by-products. NOP rules prohibit organic poultry from eating any fowl or mammalian protein.

Critics of this provision complain that chickens are naturally omnivorous and that this clause in the rule forces chickens to become vegetarians. Whether or not this is a subjugation of chickens' rights, organic producers must use antibiotic-free, vegetarian organic chicken feed beginning the second day after hatching. Conventional poultry producers are under no such regulations against raising meat-eating chickens.

ANIMAL WELFARE

Cooped Up and Ringing Bells

By far the biggest concern regarding conventional poultry is the way they live. Approximately 330 million laying hens currently reside in immense factories, each of which holds hundreds of thousands of birds in battery cages stacked one on top of another.

It's no surprise that the industry calls them battery cages, which are defined as "units of equipment connected together." (Another definition of battery—"unconsented physical abuse"—also seems to apply.) There is nothing good about a chicken's head growing into the wires of her cage; or the removal of her beak to prevent her from feasting on her sisters; or being forced to live with four roommates in a cage the size of a carry-on bag. Because bored chickens will often peck their cage-mates to death, some poultry researchers suggest hanging toy bells from the cages to keep boredom down to a manageable level. Ding-a-ling.[36]

The National Organic Standards Board (NOSB) has urged NOP to clarify the regulations concerning livestock management and living conditions. The rule states that all organically managed poultry must have access to outdoors. The NOSB, in its recommended clarification, added that organic facilities must give animals the *ability to choose* (emphasis added) to be inside the housing or outside in the open air and direct sunshine.[37]

But an NOP policy statement didn't go quite that far: "Access to the outdoors simply means that a producer must provide livestock with an opportunity to exit any barn or other enclosed structure. Access to the outdoors does not require a producer to comply with a specific space or stocking rate requirement. Neither does the requirement

mandate that an entire herd or flock have access to the outdoors at any one time nor does the requirement supersede
the producer's responsibility for providing living conditions
that accommodate livestock health, safety or well-being."[38]

"Our Commitment to Happy, Healthy, Roaming Chickens"[39]

Still, many small flocks of organic chickens exist. These
birds are free of wire cages, able to play on the floor, and
go outside for recess. While organic rules are left up to
certifiers' interpretations, other producers may indicate a
bird's living conditions on their labels: "free-run" (birds
have no cages), "free-range" (birds have access to the outside), or "pastured" (birds live outside in fenced pastures).
In any of these homes, chickens are unlikely to have their
bodies distorted by cages, but these classifications *do not*
by themselves mean their eggs are organic.

Chicken Holidays

Another criticism directed at conventional egg producers involves a practice called *forced molting*. All chickens
molt—it's their way of taking a vacation. They slow down
their egg-laying, lose most of their feathers, and for three
or four months stop laying altogether to rejuvenate their
bodies. Industrial egg producers can't tolerate chickens
slacking off for this long. Far be it from nature to get in the
way of profit margins, so as soon as the layers slow down,
conventional producers force them to molt by exposing
them to light twenty-four hours a day for a week, then
withholding all food for twenty-eight days. Not all birds
survive this mandatory vacation, but producers justify the

practice with the term *livability*, as in "livability should be in the 95 percent range." In this sense, livability means "barely alive; not quite dead."[40] The "lucky" birds return to work three weeks later. Some holiday.

Taste Check: Eggs

We poached and scrambled seven different grade A large eggs, and recorded the packing date from the end of the carton:

- A popular factory-produced conventional, 2 weeks old
- Eggland's Best, conventional, 2 weeks old
- Eggland's Best, organic, brown, 2 weeks old
- Small local producer, organic, brown, 2 weeks old
- Small local producer, conventional, 1 week old
- Organic Valley organic, brown, 3 weeks old
- Organic Valley, omega-3, brown, 3 weeks old

To our palates, the conventional factory-type, while having the darkest yolk, had very little taste, while the small, local conventional producer came out on top. Given these results, we suspect that the taste difference had more to do with the age of the egg than anything else. By checking the packing date on each carton, you may find—as Luddene has done for years now—that conventional eggs consistently show dates two to three weeks fresher than organic. If taste is your primary concern, check the date. Your best bet for freshness is to find a small producer selling fresh eggs at a farmers market or join a CSA that provides eggs. (For other egg information, see sidebar on next page.)

Buying an Egg Without Laying One

The most pressing issues about egg production concern animal welfare, and there is no question that many organic farmers provide better living conditions for birds. As with herds of cows, the smaller the flock, the better the treatment. Egg factories have obvious environmental issues, and they don't treat chickens very well. Organic eggs have no nutritional advantage over conventional eggs and are frequently double or triple the cost. If you are concerned about chicken lifestyles and the environment, buy organic—or better yet, buy eggs from organic pastured chickens. On the other hand, if you see animals as subservient to humans, then any egg will do.

EGGS DEMYTHOLOGIZED

- Shell color. The myth is that brown eggs are more flavorful and nutritious than white eggs, but the truth is that there is no nutritional difference. White eggs come from birds with white feathers and brown eggs, well … come from birds with brown feathers.

- Yolk color. The myth is that the darker the yolk, the fresher the egg, but the yolk's color depends entirely on the hen's diet. The more yellow or green (from corn, alfalfa, or even marigold petals) in her diet, the more yellow in her yolk.

- Old eggs. The myth is that conventional eggs have been in cold storage for months before they reach your supermarket. The truth is that eggs from USDA-inspected plants cannot have an expiration date beyond thirty days

from the date when they were packed. Check the end
of any egg carton for the date.

- Eggshells. The myth is that eggshells protect the egg
  from bacteria. Not true. Eggshells are porous and can
  let bacteria in. All commercial eggs are washed before
  being packed.

- Blood spots. The myth is that a blood spot indicates
  a fertile egg, but a blood spot is really caused by a
  ruptured blood vessel in the oviduct before the shell
  forms.

Dairy Production Comparison: Conventional versus Organic

Method	Conventional	Organic
Chemical residues	Use of synthetic chemicals somewhat restricted; few feed restrictions	Use of synthetic chemicals severely restricted or prohibited; 100 percent certified organic feed required
Drug residues	Antibiotics used reluctantly; all milk tested before bottled	Use of drugs severely restricted; all milk tested before bottled
Growth hormones (rBGH)	No restrictions for rBGH; limited primarily to large herds	All growth hormones prohibited
Animal welfare	All dairies must be licensed; healthy, happy cows produce more milk; access to pasture optional	Housing and environment regulated; access to pasture required

Dairy Production Comparison
(Continued)

Method	Conventional	Organic
Manure management	Must abide by state regulations; most manure recycled as fertilizer	Must abide by state regulations; most manure recycled as fertilizer; most certifying agencies regulate manure handling
Pathogenic microorganisms	All milk subject to pathogens; state-regulated sanitary requirements; large herds might result in dirtier facilities; drug therapy for high SCC	All milk subject to pathogens; state-regulated sanitary requirements; smaller herds might result in cleaner facilities; must cull cows with high SCC
Herd size	3 percent of U.S. dairies over 500 head	Few herds over 200 head

Best Bets

Dairy	Number of Current Pesticide Residues	Number of Environmental Contaminants	Availability of Organic		Price Comparison Per ounce January '05	
			National Brands*	Local**	Organic	Conventional
Milk, whole	6	6	W	W	$.045	$.026
Milk, 2%	2	2	W	W	$.045	$.028
✓Milk, skim	0	1	W	W	$.045	$.034
Half & half	5	5	W	W	$.124	$.078
Cheddar cheese	15	10	W	W	$.63	$.20
Butter	17	15	W	W	$.299	$.23
Eggs, scrambled	9	7	W	W	$.282 ea.	$.105 ea.
✓Yogurt, w/fruit***8		1	W	W	$.148	$.104

✓ = Best Bet for conventional

Source for Contaminants and Residues: FDA's Total Diet Study, 2002

* W = widely available; L = limited availability; H = hard to find; N/A = not available

** Seasonally available

***Pesticide residues are connected with the fruit. Any unflavored yogurt would be the same as skim milk.

CONSUMER'S GUIDE

Aisle 4: The Dairy Case

- Look for the USDA organic seal on all dairy products.
- Look for milk from grass-fed, pastured cows.
- Seek out organic soymilk.
- Seek out organic, *pastured* eggs.

- Buy milk from local small-herd dairies.
- Seek out milk in returnable glass bottles.
- Look for small local egg producers at your local farmers market.

- Look for rBST-free milk.
- Seek out cage-free eggs.

- Seek out artisan or imported cheeses.
- Look for cheese aged for eight or more months.
- Check the end dates on egg cartons.

AISLE 4 GUIDE TO BRANDS

Company Logo	Contact/Corporate Information	Company Logo	Contact/Corporate Information

Alta Dena
City of Industry, CA 91744
800-533-2479
Dean Foods
altadenadairy.com

Fresh Tofu, Inc.
Allentown, PA 18103
610-433-4711
freshtofu.com
®

Brown Cow
Antioch, CA 94509
925-757-9209
Stonyfield Farms
www.browncowfarm.com

Hearty & Natural
Hope, MN 56046
800-297-5997
Sunrich
Stake Technologies
sunrich.com

Butterworks Farm
Westfield , VT 05874
802-744-6855
Family owned
butterworksfarm.com
®

Horizon Organic Dairy
Longmont, CO 80308
888-494-3020
Dean Foods
horizonorganic.com

Cedar Grove CHEESE

Cedar Grove Cheese
Plain, WI 53577
608-546-5284
cedargrovecheese.com
❶

Julie's Organic Ice Cream
Eugene, OR 97402
800-282-2202
oregonicecream.com

Clover Stornetta
Petaluma, CA 94957
clo-the-cow.com
⑤

Lifeway
Morton Grove, IL 60053
847-967-1010
Lifeway Foods, Inc.
lifeway.net

Cowgirl Creamery
Point Reyes, CA 94956
415-663-9335
Tomales Bay Foods
cowgirlcreamery.com

Midwest Harvest
Grinnell, IA 50112
888-766-0051
Family owned
midwestharvest.com
®

Egg Innovations
Port Washington, WI 53074
262-284-1619
egginnovations.com
®

Nancy's
Eugene, OR 97402
541-689-2911
Family owned
nancysyogurt.com

Eggland's Best
King of Prussia, PA 19406
800-922-EGGS
eggland.com

Natural by Nature
West Grove, PA 19390
610-268-6962
Natural Dairy Products Corp.
natural-by-nature.com

AISLE 4 GUIDE TO BRANDS

Company Logo	Contact/Corporate Information	Company Logo	Contact/Corporate Information
	Natural Value Sacramento, CA 95831-2347 916-427-7242 Family owned naturalvalue.com		**Soy Deli** S. San Francisco, CA 94080 650-553-9900 Quong Hop & Co. quonghop.com **S**
	Organic Cow of Vermont Tunbridge, VT 05077 888-490-3020 Horizon Dean Foods horizonorganic.com/theorganiccow **R**		**Soy Delicious** Eugene, OR 21938 541-338-9400 Turtle Mountain turtlemountain.com
	Organic Valley La Farge, WI 54693 888-444-6455 Farmer owned co-op—CROPP organicvalley.com **O**		**Soy Dream** Garden City, NY 11530 800-333-6339 Imagine Foods Hain-Celestial/Heinz imaginefoods.com
	Pure Luck Texas Dripping Springs, TX 78620 512-858-7034 Independently owned pulucktexas.com **O**		**Soy Fusion** Saline, MI 313-429-2310 American Soy Products americansoy.com
	Silk (White Wave) Boulder, CO 80301 800-488-9283 White Wave Dean Foods silkissoy.com		**Soyco** Orlando, FL 32809 800-855-5500 Galaxy Foods galaxyfoods.com
	Smoke & Fire Natural Foods Great Barrington, MA 01230 413-528-6891 smokeandfire.com		**Stonyfield Farm** Londonderry, NH 03035 603-437-4040 Dannon Yogurt The Danone Group stonyfield.com
	So Nice Soyganic Vancouver, BC V6B 3X5 888-401-0019 Soyaworld, Inc. sonice-soyganic.com		**Straus Family Creamery** Marshall, CA 94940 415-663-5464 Family owned strausmilk.com **L**
	So Soya Markham, ONT L3R 2M9 905-948-1769 sosoyaplus.com		**Sunergia Soyfoods** Charlottesville, VA 22902 434-970-2798 sunergiasoyfoods.com

AISLE 4 GUIDE TO BRANDS

Company Logo	Contact/Corporate Information	Company Logo	Contact/Corporate Information
	Sunrich Hope, MN 56046 800-297-5997 SunOpta Stake Technologies sunrich.com		**WestSoy** Boulder, CO 80301 800-464-4246 Hain-Celestial Group Heinz www.westsoy.biz
	Turtle Island Foods Hood River, OR 97031 541-386-7766 tofurky.com		**White Wave** Boulder, CO 80301 303-443-3470 Dean Foods whitewave.com
	Udon Pride City of Industry, CA 91746 626-961-1671 Uni-President unipresidentusa.com		**Wholesoy** San Francisco, CA 94111 415-495-2870 Wholesoy Company Wholesoy.com
	Vitasoy Ayer, MA 01432 800-VITASOY vitasoy-usa.com		**Wilcox Family Farms** Eugene, OR 97402 Wilcox Farms wilcoxfarms.com
	Wallaby Yogurt Co. Napa County, CA 94503 707-533-1233 wallabyyogurt.com		**Wisconsin Organics** Thorp, WI 54107 888-299-8553 Family owned wiorganics.com

AISLE 5
Meat and Fish

I N THE UNITED STATES we enjoy an abundant supply of inexpensive meat, and consequently we gobble up more than a hundred billion pounds of animal products per year.[1] Our culture is steeped in the juices of tenderly grilled steaks, Thanksgiving turkeys, and fast-food hamburgers. But even the most callous carnivore has the occasional qualm with the meat industry. When confronted with industrial meat production, we are shocked—*shocked*—at all the slaughter taking place right here at Rick's American Café. Muckraking accounts—from Upton Sinclair's *The Jungle* (1906)[2] to Eric Schlosser's *Fast Food Nation* (2001)—occasionally expose the details.

What these books reveal are uncomfortable paradoxes. Despite our appetite for the pleasures and nutritional benefits of meat, many Americans find it difficult to digest the details of its production. A well-appointed meat counter is generally welcomed at the neighborhood supermarket, but few would want a livestock producer in their backyards. We may deplore factory farms, but we also cringe at a rise in meat prices. It's a complicated affair, with all the requisite sources of gratification and denial.

Into this struggle between heart and stomach ambles something of a compromise. Organic meat production promises to be more benevolent to animals and easier on the environment, allowing us to have our steak and eat it, too. Or does it? In what ways can organic meat address the following issues associated with conventional meat production?

- Livestock feed
- Animal drugs
- Animal welfare
- Animal wastes
- Environmental degradation
- Ethics

LIVESTOCK FEED

Before bovine spongiform encephalopathy (BSE, or mad cow disease) spread throughout Europe, the public hadn't given much thought to what animals were fed—for understandable reasons. When it was revealed that mad cow might have been caused by the practice of turning ruminants into cannibals, shocked consumers demanded change.

Despite the alterations in livestock diets resulting from mad cow, it is still difficult for most of us to think about what remains in animal feed. The adage "garbage in, garbage out" sums it up pretty well. To address the problems with feed, organic regulations prohibit many—but not all—of these questionable ingredients. What are these ingredients, and what are the implications for organic meat production?

(It's) What's for Dinner?

Since all living things are, literally, what they eat, the matter of livestock feed remains a central concern. Over the last hundred years domestic animal diets have been changed to include protein-rich foods such as corn and soybeans.[3] Despite the fact that neither crop is part of chickens', hogs' or cattle's natural diet, these additions fatten them faster. With chickens and pigs—by nature omnivorous scavengers—the problem is less pronounced, but grass-eating members of the bovine persuasion have not fared as well.

Cattle are ruminants with four stomachs that allow them to digest cellulose. Eating corn changes their digestive tracts by increasing the acid content in their stomachs. Higher acid content leads to two major problems: liver abscesses that require antibiotic treatment (see page 246) and more virulent, mutated bacteria (see page 61).

HERD WORDS

Bovid: A mammal of the cattle family, from the Latin, *bov* for cow and *bos* for bull

Bovine: of, relating to, or affecting cattle

Bull: an uncastrated male bovine

Calf: a young bovine in its first year

Cow: a female bovine with more than one calf

Heifer: a female bovine with *no* more than one calf

Steer: a castrated male bovine raised for meat

Downer: any sick or injured bovine unable to stand

Unfortunately, corn and soybeans are the most benign of feed ingredients. An even more pressing concern involves the use of cooked, dehydrated, and ground-up animals. Although the practice of feeding cows to cows has been banned since October 1997 (one of the results of mad cow disease), cross-species feeding continues in conventional cattle production.[4] But NOP rules prohibit feeding any rendered animal parts back to animals, including blood.

Cattle Profile

■ Top conventional producing state ● Top organic producing state

Total cows* in U.S., 2002	98,199,000
Organic beef cattle, 2001	15,197
Cattle ranchers in U.S.	1,050,000
Feedlots w/32,000-plus cattle	121
Total number of U.S. feedlots	95,209
Cattle in U.S. feedlots, 2003	13,219,800
Cattle marketed in U.S., 2002	11,591,000
% of cattle with hormone implants	63
Lbs. of beef consumed, 1998	26,218,130,000
Lbs. of cattle manure	2,083,782,780,000

*Total of all beef and dairy, with calves

If putting rendered animals into domestic animals' diets isn't enough to turn your stomach, try this: feed sometimes contains manure. Leave it to Yankee ingenuity to capitalize on an abundant waste product and the fact that cows will pretty much eat anything with enough molasses on it. Although there is some speculation that feeding manure to cattle may lead to Johne's disease in cows—which, when beef is consumed, may lead to Crohn's disease in humans—the connection remains unclear.[5] As with rendered animals, organic codes forbid the feeding of urine or manure back to animals.

How Now, Mad Cow

To read the headlines found on organic advocacy websites, one would conclude that we all face imminent death unless we switch to organic beef:

- "Everyone at Risk From Mad Cow Disease"
- "USDA Misleading American Public about Beef Safety"
- "Mad Cow: Worse Than You Think"

But how much danger do we really face from mad cow disease? Will eating organic meat eliminate the worry?

First, let's put the danger in perspective. Since the early 1990s there have been 157 human deaths attributed to mad cow disease worldwide. Compare that to the 1.8 million deaths in 2002 from highly contagious, antibiotic-resistant tuberculosis. While the horrible nature of mad cow disease feeds our fears and provides the media with compelling stories, so far the numbers don't justify widespread panic.

Bovine spongiform encephalopathy first emerged in Britain in 1983, when older cows started staggering about. Over the next decade thousands of cows succumbed to the mysterious ailment. By 2004 more than 184,000 British beef and dairy cows had been diagnosed with BSE.

As if devastating the British beef industry weren't enough, BSE, it soon became apparent, was infecting humans, too. Researchers developed the theory that the infectious agent was a misshapen protein they named a *prion* (pree-on), and that it came from feeding cattle rendered dead cows. The prion idea soon became the leading theory in the scientific community, although other theories exist.[6]

The prion theory led countries all across Europe to ban the feeding of cow meat back to cows. The United States followed in 1997 but still allowed rendered beef to be fed to chickens and pigs. Since then the FDA has expanded its feeding rules and in January 2004 announced it was taking the following actions:

- Eliminating the feeding of mammalian blood and blood products to other ruminants (cattle, sheep, deer)
- Banning the use of "poultry litter" as a feed ingredient for ruminant animals
- Banning the use of "plate waste" from restaurant operations
- Requiring the separation of manufacturing tracks of chicken/hog feeds from ruminant feed
- Continuing to allow rendered beef tallow to be added to cow feed

After one cow tested positive for BSE in December 2003, the FDA and USDA stepped up the number of random tests on cow brains. All of these federal actions drew criticism from organic advocates, who insisted that all the changes were too little, too late, and that the only true cure for the malady was organic production methods.

NOP rules ban the feeding of any animal parts to livestock, but they have allowed the use of fish meal as a feed supplement. The current NOP's feeding rules *will prevent* any organic animal from contracting BSE (supposing the prion theory is correct) *from its food while on an organic farm*. But BSE frequently takes thirty or more months to develop in cows, and here the NOP rules allow a loophole. It requires the following:

- that livestock must be organically managed from the *last third of gestation,*
- that dairy cows be under continuous organic management *no later than one year prior* to the production of milk.

These provisions would seem to prevent organic beef from ever contracting BSE, but in utero transfer of BSE has been observed, and the NOP rule is not a complete "failsafe" proposition.

Residues in Feed

Like many agricultural commodities, livestock feed, particularly corn and soybeans, may contain residues from recently treated crops or from long-banned, persistent pollutants. For consumers, the concern is that—by eating meat, specifically fat—we are ingesting pesticides by proxy.

The good news is that the past forty years have seen the fat content in beef decline, but it still contains enough to pass on pesticide residues. In 2001 the USDA's Pesticide Data Program tested almost three hundred samples of beef—fat, liver, and muscle. No residues were found in the liver samples, and only one in a muscle sample. Fat was another story. Of the samples tested, currently registered pesticides showed up in only twelve. But more than two hundred samples had residues of long-banned pesticides. NOP rules require all livestock feed to be 100 percent organic, thus reducing the level of exposure to these currently used pesticides, but this does not eliminate residues from banned, persistent chemicals.

ANIMAL DRUGS

It's hard to avoid the hoopla surrounding substances that conventional producers give to livestock. While organic production rules allow additives such as trace minerals and vitamins, they prohibit growth hormones and antibiotics, and they severely limit other synthetic substances like parasiticides.

Hormones

Hormones were first used as growth stimulants in meat production with chickens in the 1940s. Cattle followed in 1956. Today hormones cannot be used in the production of chickens or pigs, but six hormones (three natural, three synthetic) are currently registered for use on conventional beef cattle.[7] The FDA has set tolerance levels that are monitored by the Food Safety Inspection Service (FSIS) of the USDA.

Hormones in U.S. Beef Production

Hormone	Use	Method
Estradiol	growth promotion	ear implant*
Progesterone	growth promotion	ear implant
Testosterone	growth promotion	ear implant
Zeranol	growth promotion	ear implant
Trenbolone	growth promotion	ear implant
Melengesterol	growth promotion	feed additive

*Implants are placed in the ears of cattle. Because the ear is not used in the production of any meat products, the higher levels of hormones found there do not make it into the food supply.

More than 60 percent of all steers receive hormones. While this use is controversial, hormones can lower the amount of feed needed by about 15 percent. Some hormones (androgens) promote muscle growth and aid in the reduction of fat (the same reason humans take steroids). Overall, ranchers make about $30 more per steer with hormones than without. While this may seem relatively insignificant, ranchers sent over 18 million head of hormone-treated cattle to slaughter in 2001. That $30 extra per animal translates into $542 million.[8]

The industry insists that growth hormones remain both a safe and a necessary component of modern beef production, allowing for the plentiful and inexpensive meat supply Americans have become accustomed to. They cite studies that show that a three-ounce serving of beef from a nonimplanted steer has 1.3 nanograms of estrogen, compared with 1.9 nanograms from an implanted steer. To put these numbers in perspective, a nonpregnant woman produces about 480,000 nanograms of estrogen daily. (Pregnant women produce about 20 million a day; men about 60,000.)

Some organic advocates claim that additional hormones given to cattle pose a threat to humans who eat them, by disrupting the body's delicate hormonal balance, which can lead to obesity, infertility, precocious puberty, hypoglycemia, androgyny, breast and genital tenderness, and cancer. Because levels cyclically fluctuate in both cattle and humans, conclusive scientific evidence has not directly tied hormones from implanted cattle to human health risks. But ranchers wouldn't use them if they had no effect. NOP regulations do not allow any organic livestock to be given growth hormones.

Antibiotics

Conventional livestock production has become dependent on antibiotics for two reasons. First, administering low levels of drugs on a continuous basis helps prevent disease outbreaks among confined animals. Second, antibiotics improve feed conversion and speed growth.

In beef cattle, producers administer antibiotics before the stressful trip to a feedlot. Upon arrival, they may be given another injection to protect them from exposure to thousands of new steers. For these uses, the doses are low; higher doses are given when the animals fall ill. However, most antibiotics are used for preventive or subtherapeutic reasons.

One example of subtherapeutic antibiotic use is improved feed conversion. Giving steers a class of antibiotics called ionophores controls the growth of some rumen microorganisms, allowing beneficial ones to multiply. This improves digestion by reducing the incidence of acidosis, grain bloat, and parasites. Most beef operations see a 3 to 7 percent improvement in gain and feed efficiency from administering ionophores.[9]

Chickens on drugs have captured a lot of attention from organic advocates. Both conventional broiler and egg producers put low doses of antibiotics in feed on a continual basis—a practice that could lead to the development of resistant strains of bacteria contaminating poultry products.

While organic practices, in theory, reduce the causes of resistant bacteria, they are not guaranteed to eliminate them. According to J. Stan Bailey, a scientist with the Agricultural Research Service at the Richard B. Russell Research Center in Athens, Georgia, "there is no discernible difference in salmonella levels between free range, organically produced poultry and conventionally produced birds."[10]

Pork producers started using antibiotics in the 1950s, and the use has increased considerably for familiar reasons: to keep confined animals healthy, to promote weight gain, and to occasionally cure sick animals. Industrial agriculture's critics claim that the use of antibiotics in hogs mirrors its use in chickens and only increases the potential to create antibiotic-resistant pathogens.

The hog industry, on the other hand, insists it uses antibiotics prudently: "When a hog becomes ill, a producer contacts a veterinarian to determine the cause of the illness. To minimize the animal's discomfort and to protect the health of the other animals, antibiotics may be prescribed and administered to hogs by injection or through feed or water. Safe withdrawal periods are specified for all medications, when used, to ensure that no residues remain in meat."[11]

Livestock producers continue to assure the public that animal antibiotics pose no threat to human health. Still, the industry has felt the pressure of negative publicity and has taken steps to discontinue the most controversial uses of antibiotics.

Parasiticides

City life insulates most people from the dozens of internal and external parasites that infect livestock, so few urbanites have ever had a personal encounter with dozens of cattle grubs squirming under the hide of a cow. Unless stringent measures are taken against them, parasites can easily get out of control. As with many diseases, an ounce of prevention is better than a pound of cure.

A number of conventional (synthetic) remedies are used to control both internal and external parasites. Internal remedies include injections, boluses,* ear implants, forced drinking, and mixing parasiticides with feed. External remedies include several topical applications: dipping, spraying, or applying a paste. In conventional cattle, no withdrawal period is mandated before slaughter for some parasiticides.

Unfortunately, parasites are numerous, equal-opportunity freeloaders and can infect organic livestock as well as conventional. The difference is in the treatment. With organic beef, non-synthetic parasiticides are allowed. These include limonite (found in lemons), diatomaceous earth, hydrated

---

* A bolus is a wad of feed with a pill inside.

lime, and pyrethrum. Internal applications are limited to diatomaceous earth or herbal preparations.

How well they work is arguable, which may be why one synthetic parasiticide, ivermectin, is allowed for use on organic dairy cows and breeder stock (*but not organic beef cattle*) with the following stipulation: the cow's milk cannot be sold as organic for ninety days.

ANIMAL WELFARE

Ugly stories abound as to the treatment of our nation's animal population. Among the many charges leveled at conventional agriculture, few have the emotional impact elicited by the terrible efficiency of industrial meat production. Here as with many other issues, the size of an operation— be it a farm, a feedlot, or a processing facility—is a factor. While small and midsized organic producers offer the possibility of more humane treatment, the continued growth of large livestock producers does not bode well for the future of animal welfare reform.

Three areas raise concerns for beef cattle: feedlot confinement, transportation, and slaughter practices. The bovines we eat are, for the most part, raised in one of two ways: on the range or in the feedlot. Range-fed cattle actually lead a peaceful existence for a while, except for the branding, castrating, and deworming they go through as calves. Then things get decidedly worse. After about a year of freely munching on grass and playing with the deer and the antelope, they are rounded up, dosed with antibiotics, and transported to the feedlot in crowded trains or trucks. Federal regulations govern how long steers may be held in boxcars or truck trailers, but a few steers are not expected to survive the trip.

Once at the feedlot, they are implanted with a hormone

ear tag and fed manufactured feed. Here they will spend the last three to four months of their short sixteen-month lives putting on an additional 300 to 400 pounds at the rate of three pounds per day.

The story is slightly different for culled dairy cows and male calves. They never get to roam, spending their entire lives eating corn in crowded feedlots before becoming hamburger, cold cuts, or hot dogs.[12] Qualifying as one of the circles of bovine hell, a feedlot animal's existence is reduced to eating, drinking, and excreting. If you are even remotely concerned with animal welfare, large feedlots pose a problem.[13]

With poultry, images of cramped cages come to mind, but most conventional broilers are not raised in cages (see Aisle 4). Instead, they are housed on the crowded floors of large warehouses without perches. But broiler welfare issues go beyond living conditions. Extensive breeding for large meaty breasts and rapid growth has created chickens that only faintly resemble their wild ancestors.

In the 1970s it took about two months to grow a bird to slaughter weight. Today that time has been reduced to less than forty days. This fast growth carries with it numerous problems: skeletal abnormalities, leg disorders, high blood pressure, enlarged hearts, sudden death syndrome, and nasty temperaments that require debeaking and toe-clipping. On top of that, the birds often have trouble eating enough to keep up with their rapid growth, so they are subjected to intense intermittent lighting programs to stimulate more feed consumption.

Like cattle in feedlots and poultry in warehouses, hogs are raised in concentrated animal feed operations (CAFOs). In 2002 over 81 percent of all hogs slaughtered were raised in facilities housing more than five thousand pigs. Confined to small pens about twenty-four inches wide, the hogs' "bedding" is a metal grate that allows wastes to accumulate below. Most sows living in these conditions suffer from joint damage, leg weakness, impaired mobility, and urinary tract infections that require antibiotic treatment. Piglets are routinely castrated and have their teeth clipped, ears notched, and tails cut off—usually without anesthesia.

The final indignity for all livestock is the slaughterhouse. Numerous writers have accurately portrayed the reality of an animal's final conscious moments and the subsequent butchering process.[14] We will not detail it here. It is sufficient to say that it takes a strong constitution to read descriptions of the process, let alone observe and report it.

Welfare Reform: The Organic Plan

Do animal welfare provisions exist in the NOP rules? It depends on one's interpretation of *welfare*. Perhaps fearing that organic provisions would make conventional practices seem unhealthy, the USDA avoids specific language that might make organic production seem "better" than conventional. At no point is the term *welfare* used to describe livestock living arrangements, but all organic operations must establish and maintain conditions that accommodate the health and natural behavior of animals. These conditions can be modified depending on the species. According to the NOP, organic farmers must provide:

- Access to the outdoors, shade, shelter, exercise areas, fresh air, and direct sunlight suitable to the species, its stage of production, the climate, and the environment;
- Pasture for cows and steers;
- Clean, dry bedding—organic if it is typically eaten;

- Shelters that allow "comfortable" behaviors and that limit the potential for livestock injury.

Because of the higher premiums consumers are willing to pay for organic production, conventional livestock producers have taken notice and started converting part of their operations to organic. The NOP seems to have these new "efficient" operations in mind, because the rule goes on to say that an organic farmer can deny an animal access to the outdoors "temporarily"* if any of the following circumstances occur:

- The weather is bad.
- The animal's stage of production makes it difficult.
- The health, safety, or well-being of the animal could be jeopardized.
- There is a risk to soil or water quality.

Organic Cattle

Although organic beef producers face the same welfare issues as conventional herdsmen do, nearly all of the 15,197 organic steers raised in 2001 came from small operations with only a few dozen animals. Although NOP regulations do allow producers to dehorn both beef and dairy cows, the presence of fewer animals makes roundups safer, transportation more comfortable, and injuries less likely. Most of these steers are processed in small facilities with no feedlots and only holding pens.

Although processors who butcher organic animals may be smaller operations, the butchering process itself remains horrendous. NOP guidelines have little to say about

---

* In the case of large organic operations, these conditions may be quite normal, giving producers a lot of leeway in carrying out the provisions.

making the killing less grisly. There is no way around it: eating meat requires an animal's death.

Organic Poultry

Compared to conventional birds, organic chickens live in the lap of luxury. Although most organic certifiers require at least two square feet of indoor space per bird, the NOP rule does not specify a required amount. Consequently, organic poultry producers interpret the rule as they see fit. Petaluma Poultry in California allows two square feet per bird, while the newly hatched Land O' Lakes organic ranch provides a luxurious four to five square feet. At the other extreme, the Organic Farmers Hen House in Iowa manages to squeeze a chicken into one and a half square feet.[15]

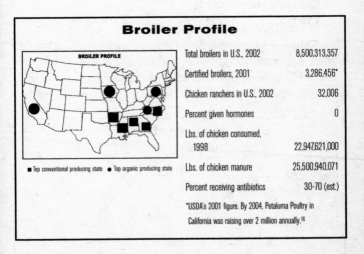

Broiler Profile

Total broilers in U.S., 2002	8,500,313,357
Certified broilers, 2001	3,286,456*
Chicken ranchers in U.S., 2002	32,006
Percent given hormones	0
Lbs. of chicken consumed, 1998	22,947,621,000
Lbs. of chicken manure	25,500,940,071
Percent receiving antibiotics	30-70 (est.)

■ Top conventional producing state ● Top organic producing state

*USDA's 2001 figure. By 2004, Petaluma Poultry in California was raising over 2 million annually.[16]

Regrettably, organic poultry has attracted more than its share of large producers wanting to manipulate the NOP rules. In the past few years, the issue of square feet per bird, access to the outdoors, and organic feed availability have caused considerable debate. Other practices, such as debeaking and toe-trimming, are not prohibited, but certifiers discourage these methods.

Taste Check: Chicken

We tested three chickens: a regular factory-type broiler, a broiler labeled "all natural, no antibiotics, no growth hormones, Amish type," and an organic broiler purchased at the Minneapolis farmers market. All were roasted plain. While none exhibited any outstanding flavor differences, there were some textural differences: both the "all natural" and the organic broiler seemed less mushy.

Organic Pork

Organic pigs are the privileged few. As of August 2004, the nation's largest organic farmer cooperative had only *eight* hog producers.[17] All together during 2001, fewer than 3,500 hogs were certified in sixteen states. Nearly every organic hog farm has an extremely small herd of

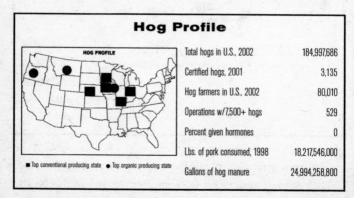

Hog Profile

Total hogs in U.S., 2002	184,997,686
Certified hogs, 2001	3,135
Hog farmers in U.S., 2002	80,010
Operations w/7,500+ hogs	529
Percent given hormones	0
Lbs. of pork consumed, 1998	18,217,546,000
Gallons of hog manure	24,994,258,800

■ Top conventional producing state　● Top organic producing state fewer than twenty hogs. Without question, smaller operations have an easier time providing better conditions.

NOP regulations require all animals be given clean, dry bedding (usually straw) instead of metal grates, so the physical impairments common in large confinement operations usually don't occur on organic hog farms. The NOP rule does allow farmers to dock tails and clip teeth, but, in smaller operations there is considerably less stress, reducing the need to perform these physical alterations.

Overall, organic production methods address many animal welfare concerns, but the NOP rule leaves numerous loopholes. As we've said before, these size-related issues can be overcome by scaling down herds or flocks. At present, many organic livestock operations are small, so consumers can be assured that most animals raised organically are well cared for.

E. coli on the Side

Most shoppers prefer not to think about the butchering process, and modern packaging helps. The only evidence left is a little blood-soaked quilt blanketing a Styrofoam tray. These neatly shrink-wrapped cuts of meat disguise the reality and possibility of E. coli, salmonella, campylobacter, and listeria.

Activists rightly cite slaughterhouse practices as culpable in the rise of some food-borne illnesses. In the end, the only thing that the nation's conventional meatpacking industry can be proud of is its efficiency in supplying inexpensive meat to a large population.

Organically raised meat is an alternative, but it isn't Eden, either. Although organic producers may treat living animals with respect and the organic processing plant may be more conscientious, organic animals can still harbor pathogens.

ANIMAL WASTES

We outlined the general impact of agriculture on the environment in Chapter 4, but some aspects regarding meat production bear further scrutiny. Manure is a major hassle for several reasons.

First, manure, unlike human waste, is not generally treated. The livestock industry currently produces approximately five trillion pounds of *untreated* manure a year, compared to one trillion pounds of *treated* human waste produced in the United States. Second, whatever enters animal bodies passes through into their manure: hormones, antibiotics, and other feed supplements. Third, there is more to livestock waste than manure. Dairy and hog farms use thousands of gallons of fresh water just to clean the barns. Chicken coops produce dead birds as well as fryers. And the hog industry ends up with nearly two hundred thousand pig tails a year. True, many of these wastes are converted for other purposes—fertilizers, feed, or leather—but unused wastes can contaminate land or water.

Cow Pies

A fully grown steer defecates to the tune of sixty-five pounds every day. Three-quarters of this mountain is deposited randomly on grazing land. This presents no problem for most of the range, but when steers congregate near a stream or creek, it can have a dramatic effect on the water.

Beef ranchers can allow manure to lie where it falls on the range, but once the steers are brought to feedlots, the manure starts piling up. While some feedlot operations compost waste for sale to home gardeners, most of it is allowed to sit before being applied directly to surrounding land. When manure piles up, it loses valuable nitrogen to the air or leaches into ground or surface water.

Chicken Waste

One laying hen produces about fifteen pounds of manure annually, which means finding a place for more than 131 billion pounds of the stuff each year. Because birds don't have bladders (they couldn't fly carrying all that liquid), their manure is more concentrated than cattle manure. Gardeners refer to chicken manure as "hot" because it contains high concentrations of nitrogen and phosphorus—and if you use too much on plants, the leaves turn brown. Due to its richness, chicken manure makes great compost. Organic chicken producers with large flocks often turn waste into fertilizer for sale to organic crop producers. Some conventional operations do this, too, when economically feasible, but more often than not it isn't. Pound for pound, manure contains very little nitrogen when compared to chemical fertilizer. In addition to producing chickens, the United States also produced over 283 million turkeys during 2002, adding considerably to the poultry manure load.

Hog Waste

When it comes to manure issues, pigs get most of the spotlight. For years critics have cried foul over both the stench and the contamination from the trillions of gallons of liquid waste generated each year by hogs in confinement. The odor from two or three pigs in a sty is tolerable, but the stench of ten thousand hogs together in a warehouse irritates the lungs of pigs and farm workers alike.

Pigs don't have sweat glands, so in the past every pigpen had a wallow—a mud hole to help pigs cool themselves on hot days. The problem for factory operations is that wallows require valuable space. Large operations (CAFOs) cool animals by spraying them with water, which is then flushed through the slotted floor to a pit beneath the farrow house. In older operations, the manure water is pumped into an open-air lagoon and held for up to six months before being injected into the surrounding soil. These lagoons can leak, break, or overflow with excessive rains. Eventually this contaminated water ends up in streams and rivers.

Newer operations store pig waste in enclosed tanks holding hundreds of thousands of gallons, which becomes irrigation water for surrounding crops. While this system eliminates much of the odor and contamination, it has a life expectancy of only about twenty years because surrounding cropland becomes oversaturated with nutrients.[18]

The Organic Answer

Organic animals produce manure just as odorous as conventional livestock, but NOP rules require producers to "manage manure in a manner that does not contribute to contamination of crops, soil, or water by plant nutrients, heavy metals, or pathogenic organisms, and optimizes recycling of nutrients."[19] Most small organic operations see manure primarily as a resource to be composted and integrated into a farm's overall soil-management program. It is unclear how well this will continue as organic farms increase in size.

Currently, family farmers raise most American organic beef in extremely small herds. In 2001 there were fewer than sixteen thousand organic steers producing waste in the United States—not a significant amount in the overall picture. Moreover, few organic steers spend time in

feedlots right now, but as sales of organic beef rise, so too
will the need for efficiency. Eventually organic beef producers will be forced to use feedlots and holding pens at
slaughter facilities. Let us hope that certifying agencies
will at least require composting sites along with the feedlots.

Unlike small organic beef operations, organic poultry
producers have increased in size and now resemble conventional chicken ranches. How they will handle waste
over time remains to be seen, once again pitting the bottom line against the spirit of organic values. Of all the organic livestock operations, hog producers win the waste
clean-up prize. For now, organic hogs are raised on small
traditional, multifaceted farms with crops, orchards, and
good old-fashioned pig wallows. Time will tell how the organic pork market develops.

ENVIRONMENTAL DEGRADATION

Fresh Country Air

Our bovine brethren also add to air pollution. Cattle
are major producers of methane emissions in the United
States. In addition, the nitrogen in the manure and urine
of grazing cattle contributes 20 to 40 percent of nitrous
oxide emissions.[20]

People can't see methane, but they sure can smell hydrogen sulfide. One dried cow patty is only mildly odorous,
but several thousand tons scraped into a small mountain
can be overwhelming. And we have not even mentioned
the stink created by meatpacking and rendering plants.
Let's just say you have to smell it to believe it. Most rural
residents aren't waiting to catch a whiff. Townships all
across the country are turning thumbs down on CAFOs

that manage to cram in thousands of hogs, chickens, dairy cows, or steers.

Where the Buffalo Once Roamed

When cows come in, wildlife goes away. Millions of cattle occupy land that once was home to hundreds of species of plants and animals. Whether in feedlots or on the range, cattle strip the land clean and leave little or no vegetation for other animals. In addition to habitat destruction caused by the herd, humans have poisoned or trapped wolves and coyotes, hunted the buffalo to near-extinction, and ruined antelope grazing land—entirely changing the western plains—all for raising steaks.

To put the cattle situation in perspective, imagine this: a marketable steer weighs about twelve hundred pounds. If the average adult human weighs about 150 pounds, then each cow is equal to nearly eight adults. In terms of food resources, having all this cattle is like supporting a population of more than a billion people. If the United States had to house, feed, and control the waste of a billion-plus people, the problems would be obvious. But livestock production takes place mostly out of sight, with the result that the public remains oblivious to the damage being done by millions of bovines.

ETHICS

Whether it is moral for humans to eat meat is a personal matter beyond the scope of this book, and many volumes have already been devoted to the subject. But organic advocates frequently raise the issue when critics claim that organic crop yields tend to be lower than conventional or industrial yields. Since most of the U.S. corn and soybean crop is fed to livestock, organic advocates point out that lower yields would be feasible if people in the developed world cut back their consumption of meat.

Although some people in developed countries—including the United States—have cut back on beef eating, increases in their consumption of other animal protein sources have led to other health and environmental problems. Such consumption will remain an issue as world population growth continues to outpace the finite supply of arable land.

TO EAT OR NOT TO EAT

These days it's hard to stand at the meat counter without having second thoughts. Unless you have been asleep for the last twenty-five years, you could not have missed meat becoming the hot-button issue on both the food safety and ethical fronts. From health concerns to religious convictions, from PETA to the Food First! campaign, eating meat—particularly red meat—is not the same ritual celebration of the good life it once was.

The popularity of the Atkins diet has altered this trend to some degree, but more and more Americans are nonetheless flirting with vegetarianism. These Americans are standing at the end of a long line in history. As far back as Pythagoras (580 B.C.E.), certain individuals, groups, and even cultures have turned against meat eating, opting instead for gaining sustenance from somewhere lower on the food chain. Today's vegetarians cite a number of reasons to eliminate meat, including:

- Religious beliefs: Several religions and a few Christian denominations have long advocated abstinence from meat.

- Environmental issues: American livestock produces five tons of manure for every man, woman, and child in the

United States. This significantly contributes to water pollution, air pollution, and disease.

- Animal welfare: The only defense one can muster for factory farms is that they are profitable and efficient. It is debatable whether any animal raised in a factory is truly healthy.

- World hunger: Meat is an extremely inefficient way to get nutrients. Cattle are eating valuable resources. About 70 percent of U.S. corn and soybeans are fed to livestock.

- Health: Though there is currently a heated debate about the amount of animal protein the human diet should contain, overeating fatty meats leads to obesity, cancer, heart disease, stroke, and the like.

- Moral issues: Animals are sentient beings and thus shouldn't be eaten. "I don't eat anything with a face" is often cited as a good reason not to eat meat.

Taste Check: Sirloin Steak

We tasted three selections of sirloin steak: organic corn-fed, grass-fed, and conservancy beef. All were broiled. None attained the tenderness we have experienced with conventional beef over the years. The organic corn-fed steak, with a higher fat content, tasted most like the steak we have known and enjoyed.

MEAT SUMMARY

The methods employed by conventional livestock producers are extremely efficient, providing billions of pounds of meat to the U.S. consumer at an affordable price. Although the warehousing of pigs, chickens, and cows yields relatively inexpensive meat, this efficiency must always be weighed against the questionable conditions inherent in the process: health issues, environmental worries, and ethical concerns. As with many of the other issues put forth by organic advocates, conventional livestock producers counter each argument. Their responses can be reduced to two major points. First, reliable scientific evidence does not currently support many of the claims about personal health made by organic advocates. (The meat industry has a tougher time sugarcoating its impact on the environment.) Second, the producers argue, the United States cannot produce the amount of meat Americans consume at the prices consumers expect any other way.

Perhaps the only way for agriculture to address livestock production issues is for the American public to cut its consumption by two-thirds or more and expect to pay four times as much. And this is just about where the issue and price of organic meat stands today.

FISH AND SEAFOOD

Throughout the last decade, American fish consumption has risen 29 percent. Fish are a good source of the heart-healthy, cancer-fighting omega-3 fatty acids Top-notch chefs across the country have championed fish as gourmet fare. Separate seafood counters line the walls of supermarket meat departments. Everybody, including the government, has jumped into the fishing boat. There are many winners, but fish and the environment aren't among them.

Wild fish populations continue to decline because of overfished oceans. Given this fact, fish farming may seem an attractive, viable alternative. On closer examination, however, it brings a completely new set of problems to the table. Enclosing thousands of fish in pens close to the shoreline is equivalent to cramming chickens and pigs into warehouses. The same results are achieved: drugged fish eating dubious-quality feed, then producing tons of feces.

A decision has been made about wild fish—*they cannot be labeled "organic"*—but controversy continues to swirl around farmed fish and seafood, potentially offering remedies to conventional aquaculture ills. We'll briefly cover a few of the issues here.

Feedlots of the Sea

Fish farming may offer some relief to wild populations, but like concentrated animal-feeding operations, they take a serious toll on the environment. The problem is that waste—uneaten food, dead fish, and feces—falls through the cage and piles up on the ocean or lake floor, decimating natural habitat.

Unlike caged chickens or penned-up pigs, farmed hybrid fish frequently escape from their prisons, interbreed with native populations, and spread disease. For example, farm-raised salmon are susceptible to infectious salmon anemia and sea lice. Although both show up in wild populations, they do so only occasionally and in low numbers. Mother Nature can take care of these pests in the wild, but aquaculture intensifies breeding grounds for both fish and the pathogens and organisms that prey on them. When fish escape, their diseases and susceptibilities go with them.

Feed Frenzy

One major barrier to organic certification concerns certifying feed. Since several major farmed species are predatory, they require animal (fish) protein to remain profitable for producers. Turning salmon or shrimp into vegetarians with soybean meal does not really work. In order to produce meat-eating fish, thousands of tons of wild fish are ground up into fish pellets for feed. In other words, harvesting wild fish still goes on in order to raise farmed fish, and wild fish are not certifiable.

In addition to ravaging wild fish stocks to feed captive fish, producers must dump antibiotics into feed pellets to counter diseases common in penned fish. As with livestock, this practice increases the likelihood that antibiotic resistance will develop.

Finally, some fish—salmon in particular—don't grow the same way in captivity as they do in the wild. Wild salmon meat is bright pink, whereas farmed salmon meat turns gray. In order to maintain the color consumers prize, producers add chemicals to the feed pellets to turn the fish flesh pink.

The Future of Organic Fish Farming

The future of organic fish farming remains uncertain. To address the issue, in 2000 the National Organic Standards Board, in its advisory role to the NOP, formed the Aquatic Animal Task Force to study the issue. It concluded that organic aquaculture systems *may* be developed under certain conditions. Exactly what those conditions are has been the subject of heated debate over the last several years as interested parties have tried to hammer out their differences. The NOP has not issued standards specifically for farmed shrimp or fish. Investors in organic fish farming want the government's seal of approval. The Organic Trade Association doesn't want organic fish operations eroding public confidence in organics. During 2003, two shrimp farms (in Texas and Florida) developed organic feed and obtained certification. The NOP let them stand but placed a moratorium on additional certifications until standards are developed. At this writing, the issue is still unresolved.

Best Bets

Grains	Number of Current Pesticide Residues	Number of Environmental Contaminants	Availability of Organic		Price Comparison Per Pound January '05	
			National Brands*	Local**	Organic	Conventional
✓Beef, steak	3	6	H	H	N/A	$7.49
Ham	3	3	H	H	N/A	$3.99
Pork chop	4	11	H	H	N/A	$3.99
Bacon	6	12	L	H	$10.00	$3.99
✓Lamb chop	6	9	H	H	N/A	N/A
✓Chicken	2	5	H	H	$2.69	$1.39
✓Turkey, ground	3	5	H	H	$3.75	$1.99
Hot Dogs	15	12	L	H	N/A	$4.59

✓ = Best Bet for conventional

Source for Contaminants and Residues: FDA's Total Diet Study, 2002

* W = widely available; L = limited availability; H = hard to find; N/A = not available

** Seasonally available

Meat Production Summary

Area of Concern	Grass-Fed Meat (Label Unregulated)	Conventionally Fed Meat (Label Unregulated)	Organic-Fed Meat (Label Regulated)
REGULATIONS	USDA, FDA, and state health regulations apply No other regulations apply	USDA, FDA, and state health regulations apply No other regulations apply	USDA, FDA, and state health regulations apply NOP rules apply
FEED		No restriction	100% organic feed only certified by accredited certifier
Pasture	Pasture grass and hay only	Pasture optional	Pasture required but not exclusive
Corn/Soybeans	No corn or soybeans	Corn or soybeans allowed	Corn or soybeans allowed
Manure Feeding	No legal restriction, but highly unlikely	Manure feeding allowed	Manure feeding prohibited
Animal Products	No animal products allowed	Animal products unrestricted for chickens, bovines restricted to fish and poultry	No animal products allowed
DRUGS	No restriction on USDA- and FDA-approved drugs	No restriction on USDA- and FDA-approved drugs	Use limited to those on the National List
Hormones, beef	No restriction, but highly unlikely	No restriction on USDA- and FDA-approved	Hormones prohibited
Hormones, hogs and chickens	Prohibited	Prohibited	Prohibited

Meat Production Summary
(Continued)

Area of Concern	Grass-Fed Meat (Label Unregulated)	Conventionally Fed Meat (Label Unregulated)	Organic-Fed Meat (Label Regulated)
Antibiotics, beef, hogs, and chickens	No restriction on USDA- and FDA-approved antibiotics	No restriction on USDA- and FDA-approved antibiotics	Antibiotics prohibited
ANIMAL WELFARE	Self-imposed standards	Few standards	NOP regulated
Access to pasture	Required	Optional	Required
Cages	Not used	Standard	Prohibited
Crowding	Not used	Standard	Prohibited
ENVIRONMENT	Self-regulated	Not standard	Some regulation
Overgrazing and water pollution	Possible, unlikely	Possible	Possible, unlikely
Manure laws management	State pollution laws apply	State pollution laws apply	State pollution and NOP rules apply
Air	No restrictions	No restrictions	No restrictions, but inspector comment possible if bad

CONSUMER'S GUIDE

Aisle 5: The Meat Counter

- Seek out organic, grass-fed beef, lamb, and pork.
- Look for organic, pastured chickens.
- Buy fish from the bottom of the food chain, such as sardines. They have lots of omega-3 fatty acids and little contamination.

- Buy meat from local small livestock producers.
- Decline to buy farm-raised fish or shrimp.

- Seek out producers dedicated to treating livestock humanely.
- Limit the consumption of meat in general.

- Seek out gourmet, limousin, or kobe beef.

AVAILABILITY LEGEND

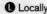 Internet, Mail order 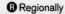 Locally ⓡ Regionally ⓢ Statewide

AISLE 5 GUIDE TO BRANDS

Company Logo	Contact/Corporate Information	Company Logo	Contact/Corporate Information
	American Grass Fed Beef Doniphan, MO 63935 573-996-3716 americangrassfedbeef.com 		**Homestead Healthy Foods** Fredericksburg, TX 78624 830-997-2508 Family owned homesteadhealthyfoods.com
	Applegate Farms Branchburg, NJ 08876 908-725-5800 applegatefarms.com		**Maverick Ranch Beef** Denver, CO 80216 303-294-0146 Family owned maverickranch.com ❶
	Coleman Natural Products Denver, CO 80216 303-297-9393 colemannatural.com		**Mesquite Organic Beef** Aurora, CO 80014 888-480-BEEF Buys beef and repacks mesquiteorganicbeef.com Ⓡ
	Dakota Beef Company Chicago, IL 60611 312-214-4991 dakotabeefcompany.com	Mike & Me	**Mike & Me** Fairfield, CA 94534 877-223-4463 Quality Provisions mikeandme.com Ⓢ
	Davis Mountains Organic Beef Fort Davis, TX 79734 432-426-2626 davismountainsorganicbeef.com ❶		**Organic Valley** La Farge, WI 54693 888-444-6455 Farmer owned co-op—CROPP organicvalley.com
	Diestel Turkey Ranch Sonora, CA 95370 888-4GOBBLE diestelturkey.com		**Petaluma Poultry** Petaluma, CA 94955 707-763-1904 petalumapoultry.com Ⓡ
	Eberly Poultry Farms Stevens, PA 17578 717-336-6440 eberlypoultry.com Ⓡ		**Raised Right** Fredericksburg, PA 17026 717-865-2136 College Hill Poultry Kreamer Feed raisedright.com
	Heritage Turkeys Sonora, CA 95370 888-4GOBBLE Diestel Turkey Ranch diestelturkey.com		**Shelton's** Pomona, CA 91767 800-541-1833 sheltons.com

AISLE 5 GUIDE TO BRANDS

Company Logo	Contact/Corporate Information	Company Logo	Contact/Corporate Information
Tiensvold Farms	**Tiensvold Farms** Rushville, NE 69360 308-327-3135 eatorganicbuffalo.com 		**Wise Kosher Natural Poultry, Inc.** Brooklyn, NY 11205 718-596-0400 wisekosher.com
Van Wie Natural Foods	**Van Wie Natural Foods** Hudson, NY 12534 518-828-0533 vanwienaturalmeats.com		**Wyoming Natural Products** Newcastle, WY 82701 800-969-9946 wyomingnatural.com
	Wholesome Harvest Organic Meat Colo, IA 50056 641-377-7777 Coalition of family farms wholesomeharvest.com		

AISLE 6
Beverages

WADING THROUGH the beverage aisle, the American consumer confronts a wall of bottled, canned, and cartoned choices. Given the fact that water is all we really need, this plethora of potables is testament both to consumers' unquenchable desires and to the food industry's ability to concoct and market. Some of these drink choices—such as coffee and tea—are older than the Hills Bros.; others—like fruit juice blends and green tea colas—seem to have spontaneously generated overnight. Since 1970 Americans' overall consumption of beverages has increased by 34 percent.

About a hundred years ago Americans' choices were limited to the time-honored standbys: coffee, tea, or milk. Coffee was coffee, tea was black, and milk was whole. Today the average consumer must make sense of cranberry-apple-kiwi-guava et al.; a plantation of herbal teas and gourmet coffees; flavored waters; and of course, those carbonated sugary treats of the soda pop family. Not to be left out, the organic industry has managed to produce carbon copies of popular conventional beverages. Are consumers better off reaching for organically labeled liquid refreshment? In this Aisle, we'll look at the following beverages:

- Coffee
- Tea
- Cocoa
- Soda
- Fruit juice

- Beer
- Wine

COFFEE

Caffeine ranks as the world's most popular drug, and coffee serves as its universal delivery system. The stimulating effects of caffeine aside, coffee harbors other health risks, from tannic acid to dioxin to hundreds of other potentially harmful chemicals.

Despite the many health and social concerns associated with coffee, Americans love it. The roaring 1990s saw a new coffee culture sweep eastward from Seattle. Coffeehouse chains and independent cafés blossomed in every available nook, cranny, and strip mall. Every major city and even small rural communities experienced a fundamental change in the variety and quality of coffee. Clearly today's coffee drinkers are enjoying a different brew.

Along with this move toward a new gourmet sensibility and café culture, coffee politics became an important issue. As independent roasters grew more familiar with the trade, they sought to redress some of the economic and environmental ills associated with coffee production and distribution. Organic labeling is just one of many such attempts. With new labels emerging, shoppers may wonder if these labels can really change the world for the better. When it comes to coffee, what does it mean to be *organic, fair trade,* or *shade grown?*

Growing Coffee

Coffee beans are the seeds of a cherrylike fruit produced by a number of different tree varieties. Of these varieties, two yield marketable beans: *Coffea arabica* and *Coffea robusta*. Most coffee experts agree that the higher-priced arabica varieties produce the tastiest coffee, each with its own distinctive flavor notes.* Robusta beans are cheaper and often are used to extend the weight of most preground commercial coffee.

Native to the cool mountain regions of tropical Africa, coffee grows on plantations in similar climatic regions throughout the world: Indonesia, the Middle East, Latin America, and Hawaii. All coffee farms follow one of three models: traditional (rustic), industrial (technifed), or transitional (a blend of the two). On traditional farms, growers interplant coffee trees with fruit and timber trees. These diverse biosystems provide a safety net if one crop fails; maintain the soil's fertility; promote healthy bird populations; and ease pest pressure. Given the high cost of chemical farming, many small traditional farmers use organic methods by default, even if they are not certified. Without chemicals, and because traditional farms tend to grow older varieties of coffee trees,† labor costs increase.

Industrial coffee production mirrors America's grain monoculture. Featureless acres support nearly three thousand uniform trees planted in rows instead of the four hundred trees per acre common in traditional interplanted growing methods. With trees bred for seasonal harvests,

---

* Coffee "cupping"—the process of describing flavors—resembles wine tasting. As with wine grapes, the region, method, and type of seed all contribute to a variety's unique essences.
† Older varieties of trees produce ripe cherries recurrently with no particular season; thus every other week a few more cherries ripen and must be picked.

the industrial model increases yield with synthetic fertilizers, often at the expense of environmental sustainability. Old-growth forest that once supported coffee trees has been cut down in favor of sun-grown monocultures harvested seasonally. This practice leads to soil erosion, weed infestations, soil nutrient deficiencies, and the weakening of natural pest controls.

Coffee Processing

The way coffee is grown is just the first step from tree to cup. To remove the seed (bean) from the fruit, coffee processors use one of two methods: mechanically agitating the fruit, or washing the seed away with water. The second of these two methods, "wet processing," involves large quantities of water that contaminate waterways. With both methods, the large volume of pulp generated creates additional waste-removal problems. Some aid agencies and co-operative development projects address the waste issue by promoting both water treatment and composting facilities. Certified organic coffee operations are not required to institute such measures, but many have done so regardless.

With the pulp removed, the beans are spread on the ground to dry before being bagged and delivered to a coffee buyer or marketing cooperative. From there they are shipped to roasters large and small throughout the world.

Avoiding the Jitters: Decaf

Not everyone enjoys caffeine's kick, so additional processes strip the caffeine from some coffee beans. Since 1906 several decaffeinating methods have been employed. Three are used today: soaking the beans in chemical solvents, soaking the beans in water, and subjecting the beans to pressurized carbon dioxide. Currently, the Swiss water process—which removes about 95 percent of the caffeine—is the only one approved for organic coffee.

Organic Coffee

Certified organic coffee must conform to the same rules as any organic crop. The land must be chemical free for three years before certification, and a detailed audit trail documents any history of synthetic chemical pesticides and fertilizers. Although these measures may benefit the environment and workers, it is unclear that organic coffee provides fewer health risks for consumers, since coffee roasters claim that the roasting process burns off any pesticide residues.

Unfortunately, organic certification does not necessarily guarantee that the trees have been grown in environmentally sustainable ways. In fact, a large share of the organic coffee now available originates in Peru, where vast tracts of old-growth forest have been felled to plant coffee in virgin soil that does not require a three-year transitional period before organic certification.

In addition, organic certification does not currently require that a farmer receive a fair price for his labor. Fortunately, several other organizations play this needed role.

Fair Trade

"Fair trade" labels address the economics and politics of coffee production: just compensation for labor; encouragement of cooperatives; consumer education; environmental sustainability; respect for cultural traditions; and public accountability.

In addition to coffee, a number of imported foods are now available with "fair trade" labels: bananas, cocoa, coffee, dried fruit, fresh fruit and vegetables, honey, juices, nuts and oil seeds, rice, spices, sugar, tea, and wine. They may not be offered in all markets, but if you are interested in purchasing them, inquire at your local supermarket, natural food market, or co-op.

Shade Grown

When it comes to coffee, another label frequently teaming up with "fair trade" is "shade grown." In contrast to typical industrial methods, shade-grown trees exist in the shadows of other trees and shrubs. This mix of trees preserves biodiversity and habitat integrity and reduces negative environmental impacts. Organic standards *do not* require trees to be shade grown. If farmers' welfare and bird habitats are important issues for you, seek out "fair trade" and "shade grown" labels. Many of these varieties are also certified organic.

TEA

Compared with tea, the culture of coffee is a rather recent phenomenon. Tea was a staple beverage in China by 200 C.E., trumping java's jolt by several centuries. By the 1700s, it dominated the English diet, and is now—after plain water—the world's most widely consumed drink.[*] An extremely economical beverage, one pound of tea can brew nearly three hundred cups. Although it has served the world's poor, tea's exotic allure has found its way into those whose cups runneth over as well.[†]

---

[*] Herbal teas are the dried leaves of any number of different plants and will be discussed at the end of this section.

[†] To set their tea-drinking habits apart, wealthy Britons established afternoon tea, a substantial late-afternoon meal featuring pastries, cakes, crumpets, and the artery-clogging wonders of Devonshire clotted cream.

Traditional tea is made from the dried leaves of *Camellia sinensis* (China bush) or *Camellia assam* (Assam bush). The China bush has smaller, more flavorful leaves and lives about one hundred years. Comparatively short-lived, the Assam bush—with its larger, less savory leaves—provides the taste in most mass-produced, prebagged, and instant teas.

Although true tea comes from just two plants, there are four kinds of tea available, each reflecting a slightly different fermenting process: green (unfermented), oolong (semi-fermented), black (fully fermented), and instant (fermented, extracted, and freeze-dried).

Seventy-five percent of all tea is produced in six countries: China, India, Sri Lanka, Argentina, Kenya, and Indonesia.

Growing Tea

All tea cultivation, whether organic or conventional, is an intensive affair—typically about six thousand bushes per acre. Because only new growth is harvested, the plant has a consistent thirst for nutrients such as nitrogen. To feed the plant, conventional tea production relies on synthetic fertilizer. Tea's nitrogen need may be a problem for organic production and is somewhat circumvented by mulching with leaf litter and pruned waste or by planting green manure crops. Animal manure is used on small diversified holdings if it is available, but the lack of organic sources of nitrogen is a limiting factor in the production of organic tea.

While some multinational beverage companies own and operate a few large "tea estates," mainly in Bangladesh and India, many tea groves are small family-owned farms. As with many agricultural products, the size of the farm matters with tea. Because each plant must be hand-maintained—pruned, tipped, plucked, weeded, sprayed, and fertilized—tea growing requires a lot of hand labor. Worldwide, children do much of that work. Child labor issues are not addressed by current organic standards in the United States.

Labor Issues

Organic tea eliminates the use of pesticides and synthetic fertilizers widespread in conventional production. But only "fair trade" labels ensure that the tea's production has not exploited children. During the 1990s it was estimated that more than a hundred thousand children were employed on tea estates in just two states in India.[1] Not only India, but all tea-exporting countries employ child labor. In 1994 Transfair* instituted requirements prohibiting children under fourteen—except on small family-owned holdings—from working on certified farms.

Tea and Pests

Another problem with growing tea is its susceptibility to various pests: weeds, insects, and in particular fungi. Conventional tea growers employ the usual array of chemicals, while organic tea production restricts pest control. Instead of synthetic chemicals, organic growers use a variety of methods: copper fungicides such as, botanical insecticides *(Bacillus thuringiensis),* and biological controls (parasitic wasps).

---

* One of the organizations that oversees fair trade labeling.

Tea Processing

Unlike many crops, tea bushes remain intact, and only new leaves are picked. Once harvested, farmers "wither" the leaves to reduce the moisture content by one third. Complete drying yields green tea, whereas fermented tea is held for several hours at 75°F in high humidity to allow the tea's natural *polyphenol oxidase* enzyme to develop full flavor. Fermented tea is then dried at higher temperatures to deactivate the enzyme and stop the process.[2] These procedures are the same for conventional and organic production.

Organic Herbal Teas

Herbal teas (more correctly, tisanes) have probably been around since humans first boiled water. For thousands of years people have made either fresh or dried plant material into tea by steeping it in water. Ancient writers developed detailed recipes from various plant materials, which have since been touted for their medicinal properties. Today hundreds of dried herbal teas are available as curatives or as pleasant beverages.

Until modern pharmaceuticals arrived in the midtwentieth century, herbs were a drugstore staple. Modern drugs did not replace herbs; they just moved them into health food stores. Several early brand names remain available along with hundreds of new labels. Since the late 1980s organic herbal teas have been rapidly gaining a market presence. In fact, herbs are often the first crop that exurbanites plant when they set up an organic farm.

The good news is that most herbs do not require the trappings of modern agriculture for their cultivation. Many produce oils that keep insects at bay; in fact, some are themselves used as insect repellents. In addition, herbs often produce more of their flavorful essential oils in nutrient-poor soils, thus eliminating the need for heavy fertilizer applications.

Herbs and herbal teas represent the organic ideal of the simple, natural, resourceful, and healthful plant, but a disturbing trend in the organic food industry is the bottling of ready-to-drink tea. Because it is at least 95 percent water (not certifiable), the consumer is paying a premium for something that often contains less than five percent organic ingredients but is still labeled "organic." Although the drink is convenient, the label escalates the price considerably.

Chai

In addition to green and black teas, chai has become a popular café order. Originating in India, the tasty drink is made from a blend of green and black teas steeped in milk, then spiced with cinnamon, cardamom, ginger, cloves, and sometimes pepper. During the early 1990s chai was available only in coffee- and teahouses, but now several companies package organic chai in aseptic cartons.

COCOA

Before there were truffles, Hershey Kisses, and devil's food cakes, there was hot and cold cocoa. By the time Cortés invaded Mexico in 1517, its native population had been drinking cocoa for nearly three thousand years. Pottery dating back to 1500 B.C.E. depicts the Olmecs, Mexico's original population, making and drinking a beverage from the seeds of the cocoa tree. Two trees from the large *Theobroma* family now provide the world with both chocolate and cocoa.* *Theobroma bicolor* is native to Mexico and is the source of the beverage *pataxte*. *Theobroma cacao*, the source of cocoa, is native to Central America, but today 75 percent of the world's cocoa grows in just six West African countries.

Pesticides and Cocoa Production

Cocoa prices hit their highest point, $3,200 per ton, in 1979, and they have been on a steep downward slide ever since, to less than $900 a ton today. In the late 1970s most cocoa producers were poor but were still able to afford such off-farm inputs as pesticides. Today they are too destitute to purchase chemicals, so their crops are "organic." Even so, European chocolates have been found to contain residues of the pesticide lindane. Further, the FDA's Total Diet Study has detected lindane in various products made with chocolate or cocoa.[3] Certified organic cocoa and chocolate products, grown without pesticides, can be found at any natural foods store.

Earthly Beans and Heavenly Chocolate

Most people find raw cocoa beans bitter and unpalatable, but a series of steps turns the beans into edible treats. Cocoa processing involves roasting the shelled beans (called nibs), then grinding them into a paste. This action heats the nibs and liquefies the cocoa butter, which is treated with an alkali processing aid to remove the bitter taste. It also makes the cocoa darker, milder, and more chocolaty.

---

* *Theobroma* derives from the Greek, *theo* for god and *broma* for food—hence "food of the gods."

After the alkali treatment (sodium carbonate is allowed in organics), the butter is squeezed out, and presto: cocoa powder. The cocoa butter is then bleached and further refined. To make chocolate, processors add back a certain amount of the butter depending on the desired grade of chocolate.

A higher percentage of cocoa butter provides a richer flavor and mouthfeel. Fine European chocolates contain 35 to 40 percent cocoa butter. Inexpensive American candy bars frequently contain as little as 6 percent. Because the organic industry consistently operates in the upscale markets, organic chocolate usually contains a higher percentage of cocoa butter.

Cocoa and Economic Justice

While 90 percent of cocoa farms are small (less than five acres) and family-owned, the structure of the cocoa industry presents serious problems at present. But these small holdings provide hope for the future of democratic agriculture. Chocolate products may also be certified "fair trade," and it makes as much sense to seek out this label for cocoa as it does for coffee or tea. In fact, it may be even more important.

Where coffee production has had its share of exploitation, it is now complicated with the more contentious issue of outright slavery. Low cocoa prices, intensive manual production methods, lax government oversight, and a lack of consumer awareness all contribute to the modern-day nightmare of slavery in West Africa. Several Fair Trade organizations tackle this issue head-on, and it warrants extra consumer effort when buying cocoa and chocolate products.

SODA

Believing that its effervescent quality meant it was full of life and health, natural soda water from mineral springs has fascinated humans for centuries. Then in 1815 someone got the bright idea to put bubbles into plain water, thereby launching one of the biggest drinking fads and most successful niches the food industry has ever seen.

For nearly a hundred years carbonated sodas were the domain of the local druggist and his fountain, because they were originally seen as patent medicines. Consequently only pharmacists could dispense the magic syrup and inject it with carbonated water. At this point the medicine found in colas came from coca leaves, guaranteeing a certain healthy zing for each drinker.* The invention of an effective bottle cap in 1892 set off a gigantic marketing battle that—complete with multimillion-dollar celebrity endorsements and nearly universal recognition of brand names—continues today.

Soft drink ingredients are still hotly disputed and the specific recipes dutifully guarded, so it seems only natural that the organic industry would enter into the fray with its own "healthy" versions. What advantage do organic soft drinks have over conventional ones? Organic advocates would say plenty; scientists and nutritionists would say absolutely none, except for the fact that the higher prices may prevent overconsumption.

---

* The cocaine—in very small amounts—remained in the product until 1929, when a stimulating debate finally forced its removal. Sodas were eventually renamed soft drinks because they contained no hard liquor.

Sugar, HFCS, and Other Sweet Things

No description of soft drinks would be complete without a discussion about sweeteners. The fact is that all soft drinks—whether organic or conventional—consist of nothing more than carbonated sugar water and added flavorings. The debate about the value of sugar in the human diet is an old one. Conventional thinking says that sugar is convenient "food energy"; traditional organicists rightly see "food energy" as a euphemism for calories; nutritionists say a sugar is a sugar is a sugar and that Americans consume too much. Industrial organic producers claim they use a better sugar (i.e., no High Fructose Corn Syrup).

The debate hinges on a fundamental misunderstanding of sugar in all its forms. So what exactly is sugar? The substance found in most home sugar bowls is a simple carbohydrate called sucrose.* All plants manufacture sucrose, but several produce enough for commercial use: sugarcane, sugar beets, sorghum, corn, and maple trees. Most white sugar is extracted from either sugarcane or sugar beets. Sugarcane grows in tropical climes, whereas beets do just fine in temperate regions.

Whether it comes from cane or beet, the juice must be extracted and then boiled down until the sucrose crystallizes into a slightly darker version of the sugar we all know and love.† The pristine whiteness is the result of further refining to remove the molasses color. Brown sugar is just refined white sugar with some added molasses. Given all the processing, pesticide residues rarely remain in conventional

---

* Once in the body, sucrose breaks down into glucose and fructose.
† It's the same process used for maple syrup, otherwise known as evaporation.

sugar. But for those concerned with the environmental implications, both conventional sugarcane and sugar beets depend on heavy applications of synthetic fertilizers, and many foreign sugar plantations still use pesticides that the EPA has banned for use in the United States.

Until the late 1970s, all soft drinks were made with refined sugar. This changed when a genetically engineered enzyme, glucose isomerase, made it easier to manufacture corn syrup. While corn syrup had existed for many years, the new method produced a very cheap, high grade of fructose. High Fructose Corn Syrup (HFCS) was born. By the late 1990s, HFCS production surpassed that of refined sugar. HFCS is now found in a number of foods and *all* conventional soft drinks.

Consumer advocates worldwide who insist that HFCS is more detrimental to health than regular corn syrup or white sugar have joined an anti-HFCS chorus. They blame it for contributing to obesity, magnesium imbalances, accelerated bone loss, hormone disruption, tooth decay, glucose tolerance impairment, diabetes, high triglycerides levels, and so on. The food-processing industry claims that there is no difference between HFCS and regular white, refined table sugar.

The good news is that organic soft drinks do not contain any HFCS; the bad news is that they are still loaded with sugar, in the form either of evaporated cane juice or concentrated fruit juice. Despite what the organic industry would like consumers to believe, there is little difference between refined white sugar and evaporated cane juice. In fact, if the label does not specifically say *"unrefined* evaporated cane juice," then it's just plain old white sugar.

Unrefined evaporated cane juice (UECJ) may have a subtle flavor difference. But despite what its advocates say, once in the body it acts just like sugar or any other sweetener, no matter how it appears in the ingredient list. If consumed in excess, any sweetener contributes to obesity and tooth decay. None of them contain enough beneficial nutrients to warrant making up more than 5 to 10 percent of a person's total caloric intake—no more than one twelve-ounce soft drink a day.

Common Sweeteners

Product (1 Tbsp.)	Calories	Carbohydrates (g.)	Calcium (mg.)	Phosphorus (mg.)	Iron (mg.)	Sodium (mg.)	Potassium (mg.)
Evaporated cane juice (organic or conventional)	48	9.6	8.5	4.1	0.5	0	60
White sugar, refined	54.6	14.1	0	0	0.5	0.2	0.4
Brown sugar	52.9	13.7	12.1	2.7	0.5	4.3	48
Maple sugar	49.3	12.8	20.3	1.6	0.2	0.2	2
Dextrose from corn	47.5	12.9	0	0	0	0	0
Honey	43.1	11.7	0.7	0.8	0.1	0.7	7.2
Regular corn syrup	41.1	10.6	6.5	2.3	0.6	7.6	0.6
Sorghum syrup	36.4	9.6	24.4	3.5	1.8	0	0
Blackstrap molasses	30.2	7.8	97	11.9	2.3	13.6	414

Organic Sugar

Despite the fact that sugar beets may be grown organically, few farmers have explored the idea. That leaves sugarcane as the only currently available organic sugar option. One U.S. company grows and processes sugar in the Florida Everglades, amid vociferous environmental controversy. But large multinational corporations in Brazil and Paraguay produce most organic cane sugar—with similar environmental implications. The organic labels on these international brands may appear down-home and folksy, but they are nonetheless owned by industrial agribiz. As with any crop grown in developing countries, fair trade becomes an issue. Consumers concerned with fairness to farmers should seek a Fair Trade–certified UECJ product.

Another form of organic soft drink, often called a spritzer, is sweetened with concentrated fruit juices.* Even though the juices are organic, they undergo the same intense processing as sugarcane. Most fruit juices are 95 to 98 percent water, which is boiled at high temperatures to concentrate the sucrose into syrup. Little of the fruit's nutritional value remains, and consumers end up paying a premium price for sugar and carbonated water.

---

* Looking at ingredients panels for many organic products with high sugar content, we've become puzzled by the number of products containing concentrated apple juice as a sweetener. Although we can't find any exact figures and no real discussion about the matter, it seems that there just aren't enough organic apples grown in the United States to accommodate all of this sweetener and the plethora of other organic apple products. We suspect much of it is imported, probably from China.

FRUIT JUICE

If you've ever made fresh-squeezed juice at home, you can't help but notice how different real fruit juice is from the highly processed store-bought versions most consumers enjoy. Commercially produced juice is generally clearer and sweeter than the cloudy, often tart homemade product. The difference is in the processing.

Turning fruit into a liquid is a multistep, highly mechanized procedure. Historically, the lack of refrigeration and preservation techniques meant that most fruits were juiced and turned into wine or cider. Except for premium wine, the quality of the fruit was not a limiting factor—including bug-eaten varieties. Not so anymore. While small local cider makers may still use culled apples, most juice manufacturers demand relatively undamaged quality fruit.

The process begins when fruit is cleaned, sized, and graded before a number of different methods extract the juice. With the most common method, the skin must be removed. Apples and other hard fruits can be mechanically peeled, but soft fruits like peaches and plums are a different story. In conventional juice operations, these fruits are peeled by soaking them in potassium hydroxide (lye). Organic standards prohibit lye as a peeling agent.

Depending on the fruit, the juice is extracted with either a hydraulic press or a centrifuge. Added enzymes speed up the process—a method allowed in organic juice production, provided the enzymes are not genetically engineered. To extract even more juice, processors often heat the fruit to 140°F, subtly changing flavor and destroying vitamins. No matter how the juicing is accomplished, the pulp must be screened to remove solids. But even screening the pulp leaves behind suspended particles, and the cloudy juice must be further refined. Additional filtration systems using bentonite (a type of absorbent clay) are also approved for organic processing.

Shopping Tip

If you prefer less processing, look for cloudy juices and settling at the bottom of the bottle.

From this point on, any contact with oxygen can initiate discoloring, flavor changes, fermentation, or spoilage. All oxygen must be removed by rapidly heating the juice or injecting it with nitrogen or carbon dioxide. Either method is allowed under the NOP.

Fresh fruit juice will support the growth of yeasts, molds, bacteria, and aflatoxins—otherwise known as microbial deterioration. If freshly extracted juice is not bottled and pasteurized, it is subject to contamination. Both salmonella and *E. coli 0157:H7* pose a threat, and several deaths have occurred from drinking unpasteurized juice. The use of manure in organic fruit production has been blamed as the source of several fatal outbreaks.

Taste Check: Orange Juice

We sampled three different kinds of orange juice (two conventional and one organic) in a blind taste test. One of the conventional juices (from concentrate) had a clear taste disadvantage—a sort of metallic aftertaste. Both juices carrying the "not from concentrate" label tasted smooth and sweet. Several sips revealed a slight—almost indiscernible—taste difference between the organic and conventional, but we both agreed that the organic version seemed even smoother and more flavorful.

Conventional processors of fresh juice have begun using irradiation as a means of pasteurizing without altering the flavor and nature of the product.

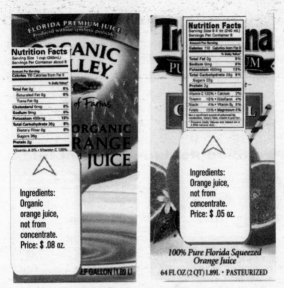

Ingredients:
Organic
orange juice,
not from
concentrate.
Price: $ .08 oz.

Ingredients:
Orange juice,
not from
concentrate.
Price: $ .05 oz.

*100% Pure Florida Squeezed
Orange Juice*
64 FL OZ (2 QT) 1.89L · PASTEURIZED

Drinking Fruit Juice

What could be healthier than drinking fruit juice? *Eating fruit.* Both the conventional and the organic juice industries have exploded during the last decade in part because consumers assume that drinking fruit juice contributes to health. Nevertheless, fruit juices consumed in excess have the same problem as soft drinks—too much sugar and not enough nutrients. (Compare juice nutrition and calorie information with that of soft drinks.)

Several studies have shown that infants from four to six months of age should consume no more than four ounces of fruit juice per day.[4] Older children's intake can increase to between eight and twelve ounces. Children ingesting more than the recommended amounts frequently experience gas and diarrhea. These studies also recommend serving fruit juice in a cup instead of a bottle to help prevent bacterial growth, plaque, and tooth decay.

Although drinking too much fruit juice may not be a good idea, organic fruit does ease the concern about pesticide residues, particularly with infants and children. According to the FDA's Total Diet Study, the following juices were found with residues:

Pesticide Residues in Fruit Juice

Juices Tested During 2001	Number of Chemicals Found
Frozen concentrated orange juice	18
Bottled apple juice	14
Bottled prune juice	11
Frozen concentrated grapefruit juice	9
Bottled tomato juice	9
Frozen concentrated grape juice	8
Frozen concentrated lemonade	6
Frozen concentrated pineapple juice	2

BEER

In 2001 U.S. farmers harvested over 32,000 times more barley than rye. While rye bread is easy to find in any store, few consumers ever encounter barley bread. So where does it all go? Into 64 billion bottles of beer. Turning barley into beer involves several steps and numerous chemicals. Organic beer is fast gaining a presence in the marketplace.

How does the organic process differ from the conventional?

Traditional beer is made from four ingredients: water, malt, hops, and yeast. The malt in beer is where the barley comes in, and its production is intriguing. To make malt, whole-grain barley is damped with water and allowed to germinate, turning the grain's starch into sugar. The ability of the grain to sprout is essential, and insect damage can interrupt the whole process. Therefore, conventional beer makers protect their grain from insects by fumigating it with phosphine. In addition to fumigants, brewers normally add chemicals such as hydrogen peroxide, bromade, or other alkalis to increase the germination rate. When the barley has germinated and the root (called a radicle) is a quarter-inch long, the grain is roasted into malt. The degree to which the malt is roasted determines, in part, the brew's color and flavor.

After roasting, the malt is ground, then soaked to allow its sweetness to migrate into the water. Other grains are sometimes added, and the mixture becomes *mash*. While soaking, conventional brewers often add enzymes produced by genetically engineered fungi to increase the conversion of starch into sugars. Any enzymes used in organic production must be produced without GEOs. After soaking, the malt is filtered, and the remaining water is called *wort*.

Hop on Down the Brewing Trail

Hops are added to the wort, and the blend is boiled in large copper vats. After cooling, the magic-performing yeasts are added. Many strains of yeast are available, each of which imparts its own characteristics to the beer.

Nearly all yeasts are manufactured through microbial fermentation, so beer is now just another item on the long list of GEO-reliant foods. Organic brews must source non-GEO yeasts.

Once brewed, beer is clarified with either a natural (isinglass) or a synthetic substance (polyvinyl polyamine) to remove all the remaining mash fragments and leave the beer clear. The final product is then bottled and boxed and ready for sale.

WINE

While the Koran states that "there is a devil in every berry of the grape," vintners might say instead that there is a dollar in every berry. Wine makers have been practicing their craft for more than seven thousand years. Fermenting grapes remains a delicate art form, even as it has become a worldwide, multibillion-dollar business. Because so much has been written regarding oenology and the hundreds of techniques that vintners use,* we will describe only the basic process and will focus on some of the differences among organic, traditional, and conventional methods.

Organic wines started surfacing in California more than twenty years ago, but they still suffer from the perception of inferiority. In addition, many organic vintners have been unable to escape the need for conventional processing aids, sparking a long-standing debate within the organic community. Given the long history and refined palates of viniculture, can organic wines reach the same high standards set for finely crafted conventional wines?

---

* Oenology is the science and study of wine, from growing to tasting.

Grape Expectations

Members of the grape family, *Vitis,* number in the hundreds. The two with the most importance to wine are the European *V. vinifera* and the North American *V. labrusca.* Over the last 150 years these two have been crossbred many times, along with other grape species. There are now so many varieties of grapes that it constitutes its own field of study: ampelography. Different wines are made by growing a specific variety, by altering the cultivation technique, by shifting the growing region, or by modifying the fermentation process.

Grapes grow in a wide variety of climates, from hot arid regions to cool mountain slopes. The climate zone often dictates the type and quality of the wine produced. Nearly every country in the world has a wine industry, but Western Europe and California excel in wine grape production. Paralleling conventional production, organic wine is frequently grown in the same regions.

Grapevines have several characteristics that must be managed in order to produce wine. First, they can grow up to twenty-five feet per year. Left unpruned, one vine would cover thousands of square feet. Second, pruning affects the yield and quality of the grapes. If the vines are producing lots of stems and leaves, the grapes themselves will be small and sparse. Third, more than any other agricultural product, the wine grape is altered by soil and climate. Finally, grapevines are subject to numerous diseases and insects. Taken together, these factors help to explain why wine production is one of the most intensely scrutinized of agricultural processes.

Cultivation

Wine connoisseurs hold that only the traditional model can produce an acceptable product. The wine industry, for its part, insists that the industrial model produces some very good vintages. As for organic wine, most experts agree that while some organic vintners are producing a superior product, much organic wine still falls short of a perfect vintage.

Traditional vineyards tend to be small family-run affairs using hand labor for harvesting. The tremendous amount of vine growth requires frequent pruning, and waste must be removed to prevent recycling of grape diseases. Organic vineyards compost waste materials for use as their primary fertilizer. Most traditional and industrial vineyards do the same, although they may supplement the vines' nutrient needs with chemical fertilizers. However, excessive fertilizer is avoided in all cases because it produces unwanted vine growth at the expense of the grapes.

Pesticides and Grapes

Pest problems—particularly fungi and weeds—threaten wine grape production. Of the fourteen major agricultural commodities in California, wine grapes rank eleventh in pesticide use. Sulfur (a fungicide allowed in organic production) constitutes over 86 percent of all pesticides used on grapes. All three types of vineyards use sulfur to combat powdery mildew and brown rot. As for weed problems, vineyards' designs allow mechanical cultivation between rows, but some traditional and all industrial operations use herbicides. Organic growers must hire laborers to hand-weed between the rows.

Erosion

In the United States, wine consumption has increased substantially in the past two decades, resulting in a disturbing trend. As California grape growers run out of good level land, they are forced to plant vines on steeper slopes, leading to increased soil erosion and a lowering of water quality. Even though certifying agencies require that some attention be paid to erosion, they do not specifically prohibit growers from planting on slopes. To stem this tide, many California counties have enacted strict ordinances regarding new vineyard placement.

Sulfites

Although all grape growers hand-prune grapevines, traditional and many organic growers also hand-harvest each grape cluster. This is important because bruised and damaged grapes attract insects, begin to mold, or start to ferment before the fruit is crushed. Industrial vineyards employ heavy equipment in a mechanized harvesting process. This damages the grapes and creates a need for sulfur dioxide injections into the juice to prevent premature fermenting.

Despite the fact that vintners turned out wine for thousands of years without sulfites, it now seems sulfur dioxide is an essential ingredient. Sulfur dioxide is added to wine at several stages for three reasons:

- As an antioxidase, to prevent grape juice from producing hydrogen peroxide
- As an antioxidant, to prevent the wine from taking on a brown color
- As an antimicrobial agent, to kill unwanted yeasts or bacteria both in the wine and on the equipment

In 2001 sulfur dioxide was allowed in organic production, but it has yet to enjoy a honeymoon, because diehard organic traditionalists still denounce its use. Sulfur dioxide, it seems, is just another one of the many processing aids and food additives that processors insist must be added to food or it won't be food.

Modern-day vintners justify sulfur dioxide because, they say, the yeast used in fermenting produces sulfur all on its own. It's true that some wines naturally contain sulfur, but many others do not. Nevertheless, sulfur is now added to all industrial wine, many organic wines, and some traditional wines. Organic wine with added sulfites can bear only the "made with organic grapes" label. Federal law permits sulfur in wine up to 350 ppm, while most organic certifying agencies allow only 100 ppm.

Shopping Tip

If you are sensitive to sulfites, look for a label indicating "no sulfites," or be sure to purchase wine labeled "organic" as opposed to "made with organic grapes."

The romantic vision of peasants stomping grapes to make wine still lingers in many people's heads, but today's grapes are now crushed and pressed using mechanical equipment that turns sixty to one hundred tons of grapes an hour into juice. The grape juice is allowed to settle, then is filtered using mechanical means or adjuvants (a fancy word meaning processing aid).

The filtered and clarified juice is then placed into either wooden casks (traditional) or stainless steel tanks (industrial), where vintners add yeast to ferment the wine. Various yeast strains have been developed to enhance different varieties. Traditional wineries rely on the natural yeast found on the grapes. In ancient times this natural yeast was supplemented with yeast from the peasants' feet. Imagine admiring the bouquet of a wine and commenting on the quality of foot yeast. (Five hundred B.C.E., for example, may have been a great year for foot yeast.) Today new yeasts have been produced using GEO techniques. NOP rules prohibit their use.

Once the yeast is added, the wine is fermented in the tanks or else is bottled and left to ferment. Sulfur dioxide is often added to the bottles to remove any oxygen.

Buying Wine

Organic wine is slowly showing up in wine shops around the United States, and many are now available online. In states that allow wine to be sold with food, some stores now carry organic wines. One national chain has a house brand of imported organic wine from Argentina.

Best Bets

Beverages	Number of Current Pesticide Residues	Number of Environmental Contaminants	Availability of Organic		Price Comparison Per Pound January '05	
			National Brands*	Local**	Organic	Conventional
Apple juice	11	3	W	W	$.047/oz.	$.034/oz.
Soda	4	2	W	L	$.055/oz.	$.034/oz.
✓Coffee***	1	0	W	N/A	$10.99	$2.69
✓Tea	4	0	W	N/A	$37.20	$12.61

✓ = Best Bet for conventional

Source for Contaminants and Residues: FDA's Total Diet Study, 2002

* W = widely available; L = limited availability; H = hard to find; N/A = not available

** Seasonally available

*** Coffee is sometimes roasted locally.

Beverage Production Comparison: Conventional versus Organic

		Conventional	**Organic**
Fertilizer	Coffee	Moderate amounts used	Some compost used
	Tea	Large amounts used	Some compost used
	Cocoa	Little used	Little used
	Sugar	Substantial amounts used	Compost used
	Fruit	Little used	Compost, cover cropping, etc.
	Beer	Moderate amounts used	Compost, cover cropping, etc.
	Wine	Little to none used	Little to none used, some compost
Pesticide Use	Coffee	Large plantations, moderate amounts; small holdings, none	Approved only
	Tea	Average amount	Approved only
	Cocoa	Very little	Approved only
	Sugar	Substantial amounts used, including organochlorines	Approved only
	Juice	Considerable amounts of oil, sulfur, and copper	Considerable amounts of oil, sulfur, and copper
	Beer	Moderate to low amounts on barley, lots of sulfur on hops	Little to none on barley, lots of sulfur on hops
	Wine	Considerable amounts of sulfur	Considerable amounts of sulfur
Post-Harvest Handling	Tea	Little processing beyond drying	Little processing beyond drying

Beverage Production Comparison
(Continued)

		Conventional	Organic
	Cocoa	Much processing and some additives	Much processing and few additives
	Sugar	Much processing, no additives	Much processing, no additives
	Juice	Much processing, some additives	Much processing, no additives
	Beer	Much processing, some additives, and some processing aids	Much processing, some additives, and some processing aids
	Wine	Much processing, some additives, and many processing aids	Much processing, some additives, and some processing aids

CONSUMER'S GUIDE

Aisle 6: Beverages

- Seek out organic wine and herbal teas.
- Avoid fruit juices containing fruit concentrates or evaporated cane juice as a sweetening agent.
- Avoid soft drinks of all kinds.

- Demand shade-grown, bird-friendly coffee.
- Seek out local breweries making organic beer.

- Look for fair trade coffee, tea, and cocoa.

- Experiment with home-roasted coffee beans.

AVAILABILITY LEGEND

 Internet, Mail order Locally Regionally **S** Statewide

AISLE 6 GUIDE TO BRANDS

Company Logo	Contact/Corporate Information	Company Logo	Contact/Corporate Information
	Adam's Organic Coffees Oakland, CA 800-339-2326 Peerless Coffee & Tea adamsorganiccoffees.com 		**Blue Sky** 505-986-8777 blueskysoda.com
	African Red Tea Los Angeles, CA 90036 323-658-7832 africanredtea.com		**Bonterra Vineyards** Ukiah, CA 95482 bonterra.com
	After the Fall Chico, CA 95927 800-903-7724 J. M. Smucker Co. atfjuices.com		**Cafe Altura** Santa Paulo, CA 93060 800-526-8328 Clean Foods cafealtura.com
	Allegro Coffee Thornton, CO 80241 800-666-4869 Whole Foods Market allegrocoffee.com		**Cafe Canopy** San Diego, CA 92191 858-271-9392 cafecanopy.com
	Arbuckles' Coffee Roaster Tucson, AZ 800-533-8278 arbucklecoffee.com 		**Café Fair Coffee** 800-876-1986 cafefair.com
	Avalon Organic Coffees Albuquerque, NM 87104 800-662-2575 avaloncoffee.com 		**Cafe Mam** Eugene, OR 97402 541-338-9585 Grower co-op cafemam.com
	Barrows Tea Co. New Bedford, MA 02740 508-990-2745 barrowstea.com 		**Caffe Ibis** Logan, UT 84321 888-740-4777 caffeibis.com
	Bionaturae North Franklin, CT 06254 860-642-6996 Family owned bionaturae.com		**CaPulin Coffee** Tucson, AZ 85703 520-623-0870 CaPulin International capulincoffee.com

AISLE 6 GUIDE TO BRANDS

Company Logo	Contact/Corporate Information	Company Logo	Contact/Corporate Information
	Catskill Mountain Coffee Kingston, NY 12401 888-SAY-JAVA catskillmtcoffee.com **Ⓢ**		**Crofter's Organic** Parry Sound, ONT P2A 2X8 705-746-6301 Clement Pappas croftersorganic.com
	Celestial Seasonings Boulder, CO 80301 800-434-4264 Hain-Celestial Heinz celestialseasonings.com		**Davis Bynum Winery** Healdsburg, CA 95448 707-433-5853 davisbynum.com **Ⓘ**
	Ceres Juices 800-905-1116 ceresjuices.com		**Dean's Beans Organic Coffee** Orange, MA 01364 978-544-2002 deansbeans.com
	Choice Organic Teas Seattle, WA 98106 206-525-0051 choiceorganicteas.com		**Elan Organic Coffees** San Diego, CA 92101 619-235-0392 elanorganic.com **Ⓘ**
	Coffee Bean & Tea Leaf Los Angeles, CA 90034 800-TEA-LEAF Privately owned coffeebean.com		**Equal Exchange** Canton, MA 02021 781-830-0303 equalexchange.com
	Columbia Gorge Hood River, OR 97031 541-354-1066 columbiagorgeorganic.com **Ⓡ**		**Fiddler's Green Farm** Belfast, ME 04915 800-729-7935 Family owned fiddlersgreenfarm.com **Ⓘ**
	Coturri Winery Glen Allen, CA 95442 707-525-9126 coturriwinery.com **Ⓘ**		**Florida Crystals** West Palm Beach, FL 33402 877-835-2828 floridacrystals.com
	Counter Culture Coffee Durham, NC 27713 888-238-5282 counterculturecoffee.com **Ⓘ**		**Frey Vineyards** Redwood Valley, CA 95470 701-485-5177 freywine.com **Ⓘ**

AISLE 6 GUIDE TO BRANDS

Company Logo	Contact/Corporate Information	Company Logo	Contact/Corporate Information

 Green Mountain Coffee Roasters
Waterbury, VT 05676
802-882-2256
gmcr.com
R **I**

 Knudsen Juices
Chico, CA 95927
530-899-5010
Knudsen & Sons
J. M. Smucker
knudsenjuices.com

Harney & Sons Fine Teas
Salisbury, CT 06068
888-427-6398
harney.com
I

 La Rocca Vineyards
Forest Ranch, CA 95942
530-899-9463
laroccavineyards.com
I

HONEST TEA® **Honest Tea**
Bethesda, MD 20814
301-652-3556
honesttea.com

 Lakewood
Miami, FL 33242
305-324-5900
Family owned
lakewoodjuices.com

In Pursuit of Tea **In Pursuit of Tea**
Brooklyn, NY
866-TRUE TEA
truetea.com

Long Meadow Ranch
St. Helena, CA 94574
707-963-4555
longmeadowranch.com
I

 Intelligentsia Roasting Works
Chicago, IL 60612
312-563-0023
intelligentsiacoffee.com
I

 Martinelli's
Watsonville, CA 95077
831-724-1126
martinellis.com

JERIKO **Jeriko Estate**
Hopland, CA 95449
707-744-1140
jerikoestate.com
I

MILLSTONE **Millstone**
Folger's (Procter & Gamble)
millstone.com

Jim's Organic Coffee
West Wareham, MA 02576
800-999-9218
jimsorganiccoffee.com
R

Naked **Naked Juice**
Glendora, CA 91741
626-852-2500
Ferraro's
nakedjuice.com

 Kalani Organica
Seattle, WA 98109
800-200-4377
kalanicoffee.com
I

 Nevada County Wine Guild
Nevada City, CA 95959
530-265-3662
ourdailyred.com
S

AISLE 6 GUIDE TO BRANDS

Company Logo	Contact/Corporate Information	Company Logo	Contact/Corporate Information
	New Harvest Coffee Roasters Rumford, RI 02916 401-438-1999 newharvestcoffee.com Ⓡ		**Republic of Tea** Nashville, IL 62263 800-298-4832 republicoftea
	Numi Oakland, CA 94620 510-567-8903 numitea.com		**Rocamojo** Woodland Hills, CA 91367 818-961-0485 rocamojo.com
odwalla	**Odwalla** Half Moon Bay, CA 94019 800-ODWALLA Minute Maid Coca-Cola odwalla.com	**SANFORD**	**Sanford Winery & Vineyards** Buellton, CA 93427 805-688-3300 sanfordwinery.com ❶
	Oregon Chai Portland, OR 97209 888-874-2424 oregonchai.com	*Santa Cruz* **ORGANIC**	**Santa Cruz Organic** Chico, CA 95927 530-899-5000 Knudsen & Sons J. M. Smucker scojuice.com
Organic coffee co.	**Organic Coffee Co.** San Leandro, CA 94577 510-638-1300 o-coffee.com Ⓢ	*seven cups*	**Seven Cups Teas** Tucson, AZ 85754 866-997-2877 Green Dragon Enterprises sevencups.com ❶
	Organic Vintners Importers Boulder, CO 80302 303-245-8773 organicvintners.com ❶	*Shenandoah* *Vineyards*	**Shenandoah Vineyards** Plymouth, CA 95669 209-245-4455 Family owned sobonwine.com
	Oskri Organics Ixonia, WI 53036 800-628-1110 oskri.com ❶		**Skootz** Tualatin, OR 97062 503-638-8822 Wild River Natural Foods wildrivernatural.com
	Perricone Juices, Inc. Beaumont, CA 92223 909-769-7171 Family owned perriconejuices.com		**Solana Gold Organics** Sebastopol, CA 95473 800-459-1121 solanagold.com

AISLE 6 GUIDE TO BRANDS

Company Logo	Contact/Corporate Information	Company Logo	Contact/Corporate Information
S T✳S H	**Stash** Tigard, OR 97224 503-684-4482 stashtea.com		**Thanksgiving Coffee Co.** Fort Bragg, CA 95437 800-648-6491 thanksgivingcoffee.com ❶
	Steap Soda Newton, PA 18940 215-860-8180 Healthy Beverage Co. steapsoda.com	Uncle Matt's ORGANIC	**Uncle Matt's** Clermont, FL 34712 352-394-8737 unclematts.com
SUNSTONE	**Sunstone Vineyards** Santa Ynez, CA 93460 805-688-9463 Family owned sunstonewinery.com	WENTE	**Wente Vineyards** Livermore, CA 94550 925-456-2300 wentevineyards.com
	Taylor Maid Farms Sebastopol, CA 95472 888-688-7272 taylormaidfarms.com ❶	Yogi Tea	**Yogi Tea** Eugene, OR 97402 800-225-3623 yogitea.com
	Tazo 800-299-9445 tazo.com	Yorkville CELLARS	**Yorkville Cellars** Yorkville, CA 95494 707-894-9177 yorkville-cellars.com

AISLE 7
Processed Foods

THE PREVIOUS CHAPTERS focused on production practices for commodities (vegetables, grains, livestock, nuts, and beans) and "semiprocessed" items (flour, cheese, meat, and milk). Here we look at foods that combine the above ingredients with additional additives and processing aids to create "value-added" goods such as baby food, condiments, canned goods, box mixes, frozen entrees, snacks, and sweets.

For consumers, these foods provide variety, convenience, and added expense. For organic advocates, they represent either the end of the organic ideal or the future of the industry. Because *highly processed organic foods* seem oxymoronic, they invite controversy. Given that fact, we will briefly cover some issues with organic processing and offer commentary on a select few sample products. In this chapter, we will discuss:

- Processed foods in context
- Definition of *processed food*
- The organic difference
- The National List
- Ingredient sourcing
- Production facilities
- Types of processed food
- Buying processed foods

PROCESSED FOODS IN CONTEXT

Food processing dates back to the days of hunters and gatherers, when fire was used to alter the flavor and texture of freshly killed meat. As agricultural practices spread, additional processing methods allowed for variety and trade. Milled grains could be made into bread. Cured meat could be taken on long journeys. In other words, the idea of processing food is not some industrial age invention; rather, processing methods today follow past attempts to improve taste, storage, and convenience.

In all cases, highly processed foods share a few characteristics and require little additional preparation. At most, consumers have to mix a few ingredients or heat the items. Because these foods come precooked, they require additives, processing aids, and packaging methods that preserve them. Thus, any highly processed food product must either be:

- Sterilized in a container that excludes all air (can, jar, sealed foil, etc.), or
- Dehydrated to the point of having too little moisture to support bacteria (such as dried fruit, beans, grains), or
- Refrigerated at a temperature low enough to reduce bacterial growth (such as fresh juice, frozen entrees, cheese), or
- Denatured to the point to discourage bacteria, or
- Embalmed with sufficient chemicals to preserve the food for posterity.

For the average American, it is hard to avoid processed food. Indeed, there are at least fifty recognized food-processing industries that make over 90 percent of all food consumed in the United States.[1] If cleaning is included as a processing step, then all food is processed. But the degree to which a product is processed puts it into one of three categories: minimally processed (produce, dry beans, eggs); semiprocessed (meat, milk, flour); and highly processed (canned goods, frozen entrees, cold cereal). Here we'll focus on some of the major product categories of the "highly processed" designation. But first we'll look at the differences between organic and conventional production.

THE ORGANIC DIFFERENCE

The most obvious difference between organic and conventional products is that organic products must contain ingredients grown according to USDA organic standards. But processed organic food is more than the sum of its parts.

Processing Aids

Most consumers express confidence in our food system because they can read the labels, see the ingredients, and decide whether to consume a given product. So are there substances in the products that are added but not listed on the label? Yes. They are called *processing aids,* and they are allowed in organic food, too. According to the NOP rule, a processing aid is a substance that is added to a food during the processing but removed before packaging; that is converted into something else normally present in the food; or that is present in the finished food at "insignificant" levels.

Allowable "organic" processing aids are found on the National List (see page 312), but "insignificant" is not further defined in the rules. At this point, it's up to the certifiers, and the interpretation of *insignificant* may come down to who is ultimately doing the counting. In the past, the NOP has overruled certifying agencies in favor of large business concerns.

Processing Methods

Consumers also imagine that organic foods are, by their very nature, more healthful and less processed than conventional. Here is where reality and perception part ways, and the proof is in the pudding mix. The Organic Foods Production Act defines *processes* as:

> Mechanical or biological methods, including but not limited to cooking, baking, curing, heating, drying, mixing, grinding, churning, separating, distilling, extracting, slaughtering, cutting, fermenting, eviscerating, preserving, dehydrating, freezing, chilling, or otherwise manufacturing, and the packaging, canning, jarring, or otherwise enclosing of food in a container may be used to process an organically produced agricultural product for the purpose of retarding spoilage or *otherwise preparing the agricultural product for market* [emphasis added].[2]

In essence, all the methods allowed in conventional food processing are also available to organic processors, and the vagary of the last line leaves a lot of leeway. That said, organic processing is not an anything-goes proposition. Within the confines of the OFPA, things get a bit dicey. Not every additive or processing aid that makes a macaroni and cheese dinner or a frozen entree possible can be used in both organic and conventional methods, and appreciating the difference depends on having a working knowledge of the National List.

THE NATIONAL LIST*

Whereas many of OFPA's provisions are somewhat rigid, the National List is the amendable part of the law. It is, quite simply, a list of substances (pesticides, fertilizers, additives, and processing aids) that are allowed in the production of organic foods. Who controls the National List controls, to some degree, the future of organics (see sidebar below and on next page). The initial National List was part of the NOP rule that went into effect on October 21, 2002, and it includes both "synthetic" and "natural" substances. The synthetic substance section lists thirty-eight *synthetic chemicals* that are allowed in organic food production. Conversely, the "natural" section lists only those natural substances that *cannot be used*. In January 2005, a federal court ruled on a lawsuit filed by an organic blueberry farmer, that 28 of the approved synthetics should be banned from organic processed food. We certainly haven't heard the end of this fight.

N-LISTED

The framers of the OFPA recognized the potential for problems with the National List, so they created a rigorous process for inclusion. Inclusion is granted or not granted by committee; no one person has the authority to add or remove an item. A petition for inclusion must follow these steps:

- First, a manufacturer who has a product or process that it deems essential to organic production must file a petition with the NOP.

---

* The National List is available for all to see on the NOP's website at www.ams.usda.gov/nop/NationalList/ListHome.html. Unfortunately it is not a quick and easy read.

- Second, the NOP gives the petition to the National Organic Standards Board for review. The NOSB gives the petition to a Technical Advisory Panel (TAP), an outside organization with the scientific expertise needed to review the substance.

- Third, the TAP studies the substance for its potential for adverse human and/or environmental effects.

- Fourth, the NOSB reviews the TAP findings, then votes on whether to recommend the substance to the NOP.

- Fifth, the NOP reviews the recommendation of the NOSB and decides to either accept it or ignore it.

The basis for these listings is simple: some synthetically developed chemicals are benign, and some naturally occurring substances are harmful. Arsenic, for example, occurs naturally in water and soil, but only playwrights would have maiden aunts serve it in food. On the other hand, a cake just would not happen without the synthetic compound sodium bicarbonate (baking soda).

The fact that some synthetic substances are acceptable and some natural products are not leads the National List down a slippery slope. Because many modern processed foods cannot be manufactured without (synthetic) additives, the future of organic processed food depends on the substances that get included on the list. This "ingredient-centric" approach garners criticism. Often a substance makes the "synthetic" list not because of its inherent merit but because it is deemed "necessary."

In their defense, food processors (both organic and conventional) provide compelling arguments for the benefits of certain synthetic additives by insisting that they:

- Improve a food's shelf life or storage time
- Make a food convenient and easy to prepare
- Increase a food's nutritional value
- Improve a food's flavor
- Enhance a food's attractiveness and improve consumer acceptance

INGREDIENT SOURCING

Of course, the limiting fact for a processed organic food is whether sufficient allowed ingredients are available to create it. For example, take organic oatmeal cookies. In the early 1990s there was more than enough organic oat flour to make millions of cookies, but there were few organic eggs, making eggs a limiting factor. This is why organic products did not start piling up on grocers' shelves until just recently. As more food-processing companies started seeking ingredients, producers began converting all or part of their farms to accommodate the demand.

Converting conventional acres to organic production is a good thing, and significant increases have taken place. But it takes time, and certified organic acres are still a small portion of total American farmland. Consequently, domestic production may not be able to meet the demand—as Americans' increased dependence on exports makes clear.

Eggs are a good example of the problem. In 2001 there were 1,611,662 certified organic laying hens in the United States, supplying both the fresh egg market and the increased demand for eggs as ingredients in processed foods.[*] If demand for processed goods keeps rising, organic eggs may have to be sourced in from foreign countries, bringing

---

[*] Conventional layers numbered 330 million.

with them the problem of reliable certification. The organic industry has glossed over this departure from the original intent of organic philosophy. If you are buying organic to "help small farmers," you may be comforted by the idea that "local can also mean somewhere else."[3] Then again, maybe not.

Eggs are primary ingredients, but the NOP has it that minor components such as processing aids and additives must also be sourced organically—sort of. One loophole in the NOP rule is that nonorganically produced ingredients *are* allowed (in the remaining 5 percent of those labeled "organic," or in the remaining 30 percent of those labeled "made with organic") if the item is "not commercially available."[4] The majority of certifiers require a processor to keep on file letters from at least three sources confirming that a particular ingredient is not available. With such letters on file, a certifier may allow a nonorganic ingredient to enter the product. Business is business.

PRODUCTION FACILITIES

Another area of concern involves the prefabricated cement food factories that house our industrialized food supply. Modern food processing facilities both large and small are highly automated triumphs of technology, full of stainless steel equipment, packaging robots, and small computer workstations. Workers often resemble hospital employees with hard hats, and the whole brightly lit scene looks more like the set of a science fiction film than most consumers may imagine.

In a conventional facility, quality control is—for the most part—maintained by the possibility of a visit from the FDA; in-house inspections are conducted regularly to prevent embarrassing problems. In addition to the usual concerns, however, a company producing organic food must also undergo inspections from a USDA-accredited certifying agency. Such inspections are intensive affairs performed on an annual basis.

Some potential problems exist with the current system. While some organic companies have exclusive organic processing facilities, much of the organic processed food now on the market is produced in either "split" or "parallel" operations.* These plants are required by NOP rules to flush and purge all equipment before beginning to process any organic product (see sidebar). All organic ingredients and products must be kept separate at all times, and the total amount of ingredients must be tallied and accounted for. It does not require a vivid imagination to envision where this system might break down.

CLEANLINESS IS NEXT TO SOAPINESS

The cleaning compounds used in food-manufacturing facilities are also regulated. Three basic compounds are used: acid cleaners, alkaline cleaners, and sanitizers. Most acid and alkaline cleaners are approved for organic processing, but some sanitizers, such as quaternary ammonia, can affect the taste of food and are not approved by certifying agents. Chlorine is the most widely used sanitizer; NOP rules limit chlorine to 4 ppm (the same amount allowed in municipal water supplies) on any equipment that comes in contact with food.

---

* A *split* operation produces both organic and conventional in the same area on the same equipment at different times; a *parallel* operation uses different areas and separate equipment.

Because inspections are done only yearly, the day-to-day organic integrity of these facilities depends on the commitment of the factory floor employees to maintaining it. In reality, workers in conventional plants may not be overly concerned with organic regulations, and the rigor with which standards are employed depends upon how seriously executives and managers take the principles of organic production.

Another loophole in the NOP rules that may bear scrutiny concerns pest control. The rules have strict guidelines on the type of pest-control measures that can be used in the processing of organic food. But it is a well-known fact in the food industry that bugs happen no matter how vigilant the control. Eventually even the most pristine and sanitary plant will find insects within and be forced to employ control measures. These measures often take the form of fumigation or fogging with pesticides. NOP rules allow split operations to fumigate or fog.

In the case of infestations requiring chemical control, all organic raw ingredients and finished products must be removed and held off-site before the chemicals are applied. Most certifiers require at least seventy-two hours to pass before the products may be reintroduced into the facility. In some cases, this removal effort is costly. Moreover, if insects have invaded the removed organic products, it would be unwise to bring them back into the plant.

NOP rules require each fumigation procedure to be documented and the records inspected annually. But it is unclear how diligently a processing plant or warehouse actually maintains its organic integrity if the only evidence is a written log.

One way to ensure rigorous adherence to the OFPA would involve surprise inspections. Steve Meyerowitz, in *The Organic Food Guide,* has stated several times that inspections are surprise visits.[5] If only this were true. The fact is that surprise inspections are expensive and rare. Only a well-founded suspicion results in any inspection beyond the scheduled annual visit.

TYPES OF PROCESSED FOOD

So far we've talked about a few issues involved with making processed products, but what about the products themselves? How well do they represent the organic ideal? While some of the items discussed here could easily be made in any modestly appointed kitchen, others don't necessarily fall into that category. For example, few people make their own pickle relish, snack crackers, or ketchup.

Consumers have come to expect a high degree of convenience from most of their food purchases, and classic homemade items like soups, cookies, and whole meals have become more commonly store-bought. Highly processed items ease the cooking burden for busy people, but this convenience costs both money and the addition of chemicals with unfamiliar names.

We sampled a number of different processed items (no, not the baby food—which never looked good to us, even back then) and reached some broad conclusions in the organic-versus-conventional matchup:

- The farther removed a product is from the farm gate, the more difficult it is to determine its worth.
- Many of the highly processed items we found were labeled "made with organic," which means consumers are paying a premium for only a few organic ingredients.
- When it comes to certain snack-food or sweet-treat items, the devil on our shoulders could be heard faintly whispering, "Why bother?" as we strolled through the aisles.

- But painting all processed food with a broad brush is unfair, and in some cases organic food producers offer more than just organic equivalents of conventional products. We applaud the inventiveness and quality of many of the organic products we sampled. But the differences did not strike us as necessarily organic-related; rather, the products offered were more closely related to conventional gourmet products.

Obviously, these broad statements do not apply to each of the samples discussed here, so we offer brief additional commentary on the following products. In addition, we have included ingredient lists to give you an idea about what you are (and are not) getting in your processed food by purchasing organic.

Baby Food

What to feed the little ones is a delicate issue that falls outside the realm of this book. As we discussed in Chapter 3, concerns about pesticide residues in the diets of infants and children are a serious issue for both mothers and society.

If you have ever questioned the danger of chemicals in baby food, you are probably already buying organic, but if you are still wondering about whether to buy organic baby food, the facts in the case are simple (although the interpretation is not).

According to the 2003 Total Diet Study, the conventional baby foods tested contained trace amounts of various pesticides—some more than others. For example, those including meat had slightly higher residues of the DDT breakdown product DDE. Although no organic baby foods were tested, it is safe to assume that they would also contain this persistent residue. On a more positive note, many of the other residues found do not come from banned, persistent substances, so it may be true that organics offer a safer alternative—but that does not guarantee that they will be pesticide free.

As for other differences, the ingredient list speaks for itself:

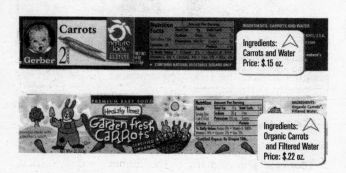

Condiments

Condiments are another class of processed foods that few people bother to make at home; most of us won't bother to buy the raw ingredients and fire up the Cuisinart. Therefore, deciding whether to purchase the organic equivalent comes down to the ingredient lists, price, and—perhaps—the belief that you are contributing in some small way to the further expansion of the organic food sector. As for the contents and the processing methods, they are identical except for the certified ingredients and the absence of High Fructose Corn Syrup in the organic version.

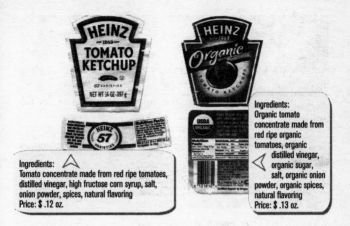

Ingredients:
Tomato concentrate made from red ripe tomatoes,
distilled vinegar, high fructose corn syrup, salt,
onion powder, spices, natural flavoring
Price: $ .12 oz.

Ingredients:
Organic tomato
concentrate made from
red ripe organic
tomatoes, organic
distilled vinegar,
organic sugar,
salt, organic onion
powder, organic spices,
natural flavoring
Price: $ .13 oz.

Canned Goods

While we couldn't tell the difference between organic
and conventional in many of the canned beans we tried,
soups are another matter. Here some distinctions can be
made. The addition of cream to the organic version certainly makes for a thicker, richer, more gourmetlike soup
(the reason for the wheat flour in the conventional), but it
also adds some fat to the mix. As with all organic products,
sweetness is provided by sugar, not by corn syrup. And the
ingredient list is slightly shorter, eschewing the addition of
the tangy citric acid (although it is allowed in organics)
and the color preservative ascorbic acid (which is also allowed).

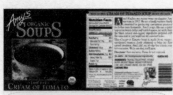

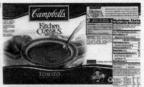

No GMOs - No Bioengineered Ingredients
Ingredients:
Organic Tomato Puree, Filtered Water, Organic Cream, Organic Evaporated Cane Juice, Organic Onions, Sea Salt, Spices
Price: $ .10 oz.

Ingredients:
Tomato Puree (water, tomato paste), Water, High Fructose Corn Syrup, Wheat Flour, Salt, Flavoring, Citric Acid, Ascorbic Acid (added to help retain color)
Price: $ .08 oz.

Boxed Mixes

One of the most popular packaged products since 1947, macaroni and cheese soon found its way into organic food companies' product lines, and boxes of it now fill whole shelves of natural food stores and supermarkets. Here as with many equivalent products, organic producers offer a slightly wider variety of possibilities, but we chose

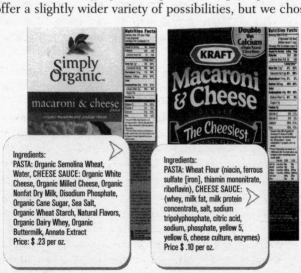

Ingredients:
PASTA: Organic Semolina Wheat, Water, CHEESE SAUCE: Organic White Cheese, Organic Milled Cheese, Organic Nonfat Dry Milk, Disodium Phosphate, Organic Cane Sugar, Sea Salt, Organic Wheat Starch, Natural Flavors, Organic Dairy Whey, Organic Buttermilk, Annato Extract
Price: $ .23 per oz.

Ingredients:
PASTA: Wheat Flour (niacin, ferrous sulfate [iron], thiamin mononitrate, riboflavin), CHEESE SAUCE: (whey, milk fat, milk protein concentrate, salt, sodium tripolyphosphate, citric acid, sodium, phosphate, yellow 5, yellow 6, cheese culture, enzymes)
Price $ .10 per oz.

to compare the standard orange-colored variety. The distinctive color of classic boxed mac and cheese comes from the approved substance annatto extract, while conventional products use the less exotically named color/number combinations we've all come to appreciate over the years.

As for the other ingredients, the organic pasta is not enriched, and the sea salt (no flowing agent) makes a predictable appearance. While some differences exist in the cheese sauce (the different phosphates perform the same function), our palates are not refined enough to tell the difference. Perhaps it has something to do with the fact that all brands use dehydration as the preservation method, or that they all manage to turn cheese into something that fits into those little envelopes.

Frozen Entrees

We have now reached the level of processing that requires a Ph.D.—or at least an appreciation for the poetry of modern chemistry—to comprehend. Perhaps the first line says it all. With organic dinners you get "cooked," "fresh" pasta, whereas conventional dinners offers only a "product." The list continues in much the same manner. The organic dinner package offers a highly readable, even simple ingredient list—refreshingly direct. The conventional version, on the other hand, makes stylized obtuseness a badge of honor. (Hydrolyzed beef protein, anyone?)

To be fair, when you really break down the list of the conventional ingredients, the differences aren't all that great, but the addition of two types of dextrin and gum arabic is a good indication that the product requires a good bit of firming up—something to hold it all together. The absence of these chemicals in the organic dinner gives it a more gourmet, just-made-recently feel. Another concern for some shoppers may be the differences in oil. The partially

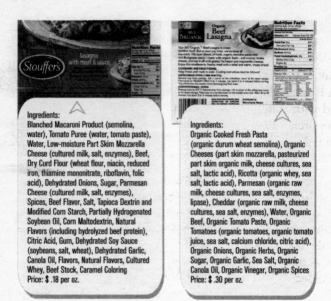

Ingredients:
Blanched Macaroni Product (semolina, water), Tomato Puree (water, tomato paste), Water, Low-moisture Part Skim Mozzarella Cheese (cultured milk, salt, enzymes), Beef, Dry Curd Flour (wheat flour, niacin, reduced iron, thiamine mononitrate, riboflavin, folic acid), Dehydrated Onions, Sugar, Parmesan Cheese (cultured milk, salt, enzymes), Spices, Beef Flavor, Salt, Tapioca Dextrin and Modified Corn Starch, Partially Hydrogenated Soybean Oil, Corn Maltodextrin, Natural Flavors (including hydrolyzed beef protein), Citric Acid, Gum, Dehydrated Soy Sauce (soybeans, salt, wheat), Dehydrated Garlic, Canola Oil, Flavors, Natural Flavors, Cultured Whey, Beef Stock, Caramel Coloring
Price: $ .18 per oz.

Ingredients:
Organic Cooked Fresh Pasta (organic durum wheat semolina), Organic Cheeses (part skim mozzarella, pasteurized part skim organic milk, cheese cultures, sea salt, lactic acid), Ricotta (organic whey, sea salt, lactic acid), Parmesan (organic raw milk, cheese cultures, sea salt, enzymes, lipase), Cheddar (organic raw milk, cheese cultures, sea salt, enzymes), Water, Organic Beef, Organic Tomato Paste, Organic Tomatoes (organic tomatoes, organic tomato juice, sea salt, calcium chloride, citric acid), Organic Onions, Organic Herbs, Organic Sugar, Organic Garlic, Sea Salt, Organic Canola Oil, Organic Vinegar, Organic Spices
Price: $ .30 per oz.

hydrogenated oil found in the conventional dinner is a polyunsaturated, linoleic acid and therefore is not currently considered to be quite as healthy. But the organic brand contains more fat and calories in a smaller serving size.

Snacks

Although snacks are easier to dismiss as an important organic purchase, some meaningful differences may exist among them. If it's chips you're after, the differences will be less noticeable (especially when organic chips are compared to the "gourmet" chips they most closely resemble). Pay close attention to the packaging. Most likely you'll find "made with organic" on the label. Again, you are paying a premium price for a few organic ingredients.

Organic snack crackers are slightly more healthful (noticeable in terms of taste and mouthfeel), since hydrogenated oils are replaced by those higher in oleic acid. Other than the oil, the only other significant difference between organic and conventional snack crackers is the inclusion of High Fructose Corn Syrup in conventional crackers.

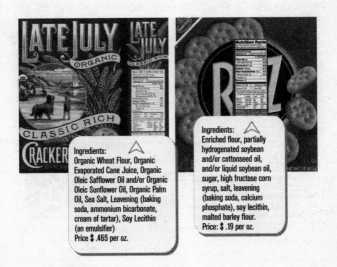

Ingredients:
Organic Wheat Flour, Organic Evaporated Cane Juice, Organic Oleic Safflower Oil and/or Organic Oleic Sunflower Oil, Organic Palm Oil, Sea Salt, Leavening (baking soda, ammonium bicarbonate, cream of tartar), Soy Lecithin (an emulsifier)
Price $ .465 per oz.

Ingredients:
Enriched flour, partially hydrogenated soybean and/or cottonseed oil, and/or liquid soybean oil, sugar, high fructose corn syrup, salt, leavening (baking soda, calcium phosphate), soy lecithin, malted barley flour.
Price: $ .19 per oz.

Sweets

We have nothing against a treat now and then, but Newman's amusing, self-deprecating marketing tagline, "shameless exploitation in the pursuit of good," captures the essence of organic sweets. After sampling the sandwich cookies and toaster pastries, we had a hard time feeling organic. There's just something about white crème filling and sweet, gooey apple stuff that defies the label. Nevertheless, there are quality organic sweets out there.

If resemblance to something from Grandma's kitchen is used as a criterion for evaluating organic processed foods, then oatmeal raisin cookies come close. The ingredient list for these cookies reveals some of the trademarks of highly processed organic food: evaporated cane juice (sugar), oleic oils, and sea salt. In addition, the organic *oatmeal* cookies we sampled actually contained rolled oats as their first ingredient, quite an achievement considering the conventional equivalent.

For what it's worth, these cookies were very good and carefully packaged, but they were quite a bit more expensive than the conventional brand. We couldn't help but think that if you're going to spend the dough, take a little extra time to pull some fresh cookies out of the oven.

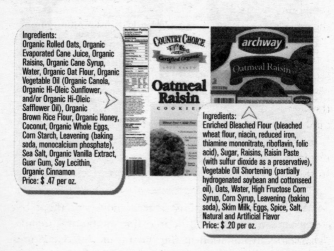

Ingredients:
Organic Rolled Oats, Organic Evaporated Cane Juice, Organic Raisins, Organic Cane Syrup, Water, Organic Oat Flour, Organic Vegetable Oil (Organic Canola, Organic Hi-Oleic Sunflower, and/or Organic Hi-Oleic Safflower Oil), Organic Brown Rice Flour, Organic Honey, Coconut, Organic Whole Eggs, Corn Starch, Leavening (baking soda, monocalcium phosphate), Sea Salt, Organic Vanilla Extract, Guar Gum, Soy Lecithin, Organic Cinnamon
Price: $ .47 per oz.

Ingredients:
Enriched Bleached Flour (bleached wheat flour, niacin, reduced iron, thiamine mononitrate, riboflavin, folic acid), Sugar, Raisins, Raisin Paste (with sulfur dioxide as a preservative), Vegetable Oil Shortening (partially hydrogenated soybean and cottonseed oil), Oats, Water, High Fructose Corn Syrup, Corn Syrup, Leavening (baking soda), Skim Milk, Eggs, Spice, Salt, Natural and Artificial Flavor
Price: $ .20 per oz.

BUYING PROCESSED FOODS

Deciding whether to buy highly processed organic products puts you at the heart of the debate over the soul and

future of organics. If the purpose of organics is to constitute a different type of agricultural system, the processing
of food blurs the distinction between organic and conventional. Kate Clancy and Fred Kirschenmann, in a 1999 es-
say, forcefully argue that "processing which fails to retain
the original integrity of the food produced on organic
farms should no longer be labeled as organic food."[6]

The problem boils down to a distinction between food
production and food processing. While the NOP rule sets
clear guidelines for how organic food can be grown and
raised, it has left the regulation of processing open to
interpretation—and for good (economic) reasons. Consumers demand processed foods, and the continued expansion of the organic food sector could very well depend on
the ability of organic food companies to produce more of
the processed items consumers want.

Your decision to buy (or not to buy) highly processed
food directly affects the supply of these items and the
food-production practices that create the ingredients. If
you value the production practices discussed in Aisles 1
through 6, buying food that contains those products certainly will encourage the growth of that supply.

But the continued expansion of highly processed product lines will continue to exert pressure on the NOP to
further weaken standards, diluting the "differentiation" so
important to maintaining the integrity of organics. If you
buy an organic Twinkie, does it really taste *organic*? Do
highly processed foods—much as we Americans love and
depend on them—really reflect the values of wholeness
contained in the very word *organic*?

Of course, this is a decision only you can make each
week, aisle to aisle. Keeping in mind that some processed
foods are more "necessary" than others, we respectfully
encourage you to buy "nearer to the farm gate." That is,

the closer you can bring your purchases to the location and spirit of the natural, the more valuable (and ironically, the cheaper) they become.

Best Bets

Processed Foods	Number of Current Pesticide Residues	Number of Environmental Contaminants	Availability of Organic		Price Comparison Per Pound January '05	
			National Brands*	Local**	Organic	Conventional
✓Tomato Soup	4	0	W	L	S.10	S.08
✓Cereal	7	1	W	L	S.21	S.27
Crackers	16	6	W	L	S.46	S.19
Cookies	21	6	W	L	S.47	S.20
Lasagna	10	4	W	L	S.30	S.30
Ketchup	17	1	W	L	S.13	S.12
Baby Food, Carrots	6	5	W	L	S.22	S.15
✓Macaroni & Cheese	4	4	W	L	S.17	S.11

✓ = Best Bet for conventional

Source for Contaminants and Residues: FDA's Total Diet Study, 2002

* W=widely available; L=limited availability; H=hard to find; N/A=not available

** Seasonally available

CONSUMER'S GUIDE

Aisle 7: Processed Foods

- Become an avid label reader.
- Avoid products with long ingredient lists.
- Choose less processed over more processed (for example, canned vegetable soup over corn chips).

- Seek out products with less packaging.
- Seek out products in recyclable packaging.

- Look for socially conscious companies with liberal charity projects.
- Seek out brands using Fair Trade products.
- Look for family-owned companies.

- Seek gourmet items.
- Look for specials.

AVAILABILITY LEGEND

 Internet, Mail order  Locally ® Regionally ⑤ Statewide

AISLE 7 GUIDE TO BRANDS

Company Logo	Contact/Corporate Information	Company Logo	Contact/Corporate Information

Adrienne's Gourmet Foods
Santa Barbara, CA 93111
805-964-6848
adriennes.com

Bella Vista Farm, Inc.
Lawton, OK 73505
866-BESTJAM
Family owned
bellavistafarm.com

Ah!Laska
San Leandro, CA 94577
907-235-2673
nSpired Natural Foods
nspiredfoods.com

Bionaturae
North Franklin, CT 06254
860-642-6996
Family owned
bionaturae.com

AllGoode Organics
Santa Barbara, CA 93160
888-980-8884
allgoodeorganics.com

Bisca
Paramus, NJ 07652
201-909-0808
International Foods
internaturalfoods.com

Amy's Kitchen
Petaluma, CA 94953
707-578-7188
Independently owned
amys.com

Blueberry Hill Organics
N. Kingstown, RI 02852
888-598-2444
blueberryhillorganics.com

Annie's Homegrown
Wakefield, MA 01880
781-224-1172
Annie's Homegrown, Inc.
annies.com

Bob's Red Mill
Milwaukie, OR 97222
800-553-2258
Bob's Red Mill Natural Foods
bobsredmill.com

Annie's Naturals
North Calais, VT 05670
802-456-8866
anniesnaturals.com

Boca Burger
800-422-6950
Kraft
Altria (Philip Morris)
bocaburger.com

Barbara's Bakery
Petaluma, CA 94954
707-765-2273
barbarasbakery.com

Breadshop
Boulder, CO 80301
800-434-4246
Hain-Celestial
Heinz
www.hain-celestial.com

Bearitos
Little Bear Organics
Garden City, NY 11530
800-434-4246
Hain-Celestial
Heinz
westbrae.com

C & H
Crockett, CA 94525
925-688-1722
C & H Sugar
candhsugarcompany.com

AISLE 7 GUIDE TO BRANDS

Company Logo	Contact/Corporate Information	Company Logo	Contact/Corporate Information

Casbah
Casbah Sahara
Boulder, CO 80301
800-434-4246
Hain-Celestial
Heinz
www.hain-celestial.com

Drew's All Natural
Greenfield, MA 01301
413-773-3739
chefdrew.com

Cascadian Farm
Sedro-Woolley, WA 98284
800-624-4123
Small Planet Foods
General Mills
cfarm.com

Earth's Best
Boulder, CO 80301
800-434-4246
Hain-Celestial
Heinz
earthsbest.com

Cedarlane Foods
Carson, CA 90746
310-886-7720
cedarlanefoods.com

Echoes of Summer
West Chatham, MA 02669
262-763-9551
Family owned
echoesofsummer.com

Country Choice
Eden Prairie, MN 55344
952-829-8824
countrychoicenaturals.com

Eden Foods
Clinton, MI 49236
888-424-EDEN
Independently owned
eden-foods.com

Crofters
Parry Sound, ONT P2A 2X8
705-746-6301
Clement Pappas
croftersorganic.com

Edward & Sons
Carpinteria, CA 93014
805-684-8500
Edward & Sons Trading Co.
edwardandsons.com

DeBoles
Boulder, CO 80301
800-434-4246
Hain-Celestial
Heinz
www.hain-celestial.com

Endangered Species
Talent, OR 97540
541-535-2170
chocolatebar.com

Dr. Kracker
Dallas, TX 75238
214-503-1971
drkracker.com

Enrico's
Syracuse, NY 13206
888-472-8237
Ventre Packing Co.
enricos.com

Dr. Oetker
Mississauga, ONT L5S 1E5
905-678-1311
oetker.com

Envirokidz
Blaine, WA 98230
604-248-8777
Nature's Path Foods
envirokidz.com

AISLE 7 GUIDE TO BRANDS

Company Logo	Contact/Corporate Information	Company Logo	Contact/Corporate Information
	Fiddler's Green Farm Belfast, ME 04915 800-729-7935 Family owned fiddlersgreenfarm.com		**Green & Black's** Portsmouth, RI 02871 800-848-1128 greenandblacks.com
	Flavorganics Newark, NJ 07105 973-344-8014 flavorganics.com		**Hain** Garden City, NY 11530 800-434-4246 Hain-Celestial Heinz hainpurefoods.com
	Frog Hollow Farm Brentwood, CA 94513 888-779-4511 Independently owned froghollow.com		**Harvest Sun** Acton, ONT L7J 2L7 519-853-3899 Anke Kruse Organics ankekruseorganics.com
	Frontera Chicago , IL 800-509-4441 Frontera Foods fronterakitchens.com		**Health Valley** Boulder, CO 80301 800-434-4246 Hain-Celestial Heinz hain-celestial.com
	Frutti di Bosco Boulder, CO 80301 800-434-4246 Hain-Celestial Heinz hain-celestial.com		**Heinz Organic** Heinz heinz.com
	Gaeta 800-669-2681 Gaeta Imports gaetaimports.com		**Imagine Foods** Garden City, NY 11530 800-333-6339 Hain-Celestial Heinz imaginefoods.com
	Gardenburger Clearfield, UT 84016 800-459-7079 Gardenburger Authentic Foods Co. gardenburger.com		**Immaculate Baking Co.** Hendersonville, NC 28792 828-696-1655 immaculatebaking.com
	Garden of Eatin' Mellville, NY 11747 631-720-2200 Hain-Celestial / Heinz gardenofeatin.com		**Island Organics** Honoka'a, HI 96727 808-775-8115 Family owned islandorganics.com

AISLE 7 GUIDE TO BRANDS

Company Logo	Contact/Corporate Information	Company Logo	Contact/Corporate Information
	Jubilee Chocolates Philadelphia, PA 93609-1112 215-386-3860 jubileechocolates.com		**Lowell Farms** El Campo, TX 77437 979-543-4950 lowellfarms.com ❶
	June Taylor Jams Oakland, CA 94608 570-923-1522 June Taylor Company junetaylorjams.com ❶		**Lundberg Family Farm** Richvale, CA 95974 530-882-4551 Family owned lundberg.com
	Kettle Foods Salem, OR 97308 888-4-KETTLE Kettle Foods kettlefoods.com		**Mediterranean Organic** Katonah, NY 10536 914-232-3102 mediterraneanorganic.com
	Lagier Ranches Escalon, CA 95320 209-982-5618 Lagier Ranches lagierranches.com ❶		**Mojo Jerky** Madison, WI 53703 608-255-2002 USA Organics mojojerky.com
	Late July Hyannis, MA 02601 508-775-1221 Cape Cod Potato Chips latejuly.com	Monari Federzoni	**Monari Federzoni** Paramus, NJ 07652 201-909-0808 Internatural Foods internaturalfoods.com
	Leroux Creek Foods Hotchkiss, CO 81419 970-872-2256 lerouxcreek.com		**Moosewood** Brockton, MA 02301 877-400-5997 Fairfield Farm Kitchens fairfieldfarmkitchens.com
	Let's Do . . . Organic Carpinteria, CA 93014 805-684-8500 Edward & Sons Trading Co. edwardandsons.com		**Mori-Nu** Torrance, CA 90501 310-787-0200 Morinaga Nutritional Foods morinu.com
	Long Grove Confectionery Co. Buffalo Grove, IL 60089 800-373-3102 longgrove.com	Morningstar Farms	**Morningstar Farms** Battle Creek, MI 49016 800-557-6525 Worthington Foods, Inc. Kellogg's morningstarfarms.com

AISLE 7 GUIDE TO BRANDS

Company Logo	Contact/Corporate Information	Company Logo	Contact/Corporate Information
	Muir Glen Sedro-Woolley, WA 98284 800-832-6345 Cascadian Farms Small Planet Foods / General Mills Cfarm.com	**Nile** spice	**Nile Spice** Boulder, CO 80301 800-434-4246 Hain-Celestial Heinz hain-celestial.com
Nasoya	**Nasoya** Ayer, MA 01432 800-229-8638 Vitasoy, Inc. Vitasoy International Holdings nasoya.com		**Noble Harvest Food Company** Jupiter, FL 33478 nobleharvestfood.com
NATIVE FOREST	**Native Forest** Carpinteria, CA 93014 805-684-8500 Edward & Sons Trading Co. edwardandsons.com		**Nuevo Latino Food Co.** Boulder, CO 303-564-8848 nuevolatinofood.com
Natural Value	**Natural Value** Sacramento, CA 95831-2347 916-427-7242 Family owned naturalvalue.com	**CLASSICS**	**Organic Classics** Brockton, MA 02301 877-400-5997 Fairfield Farm Kitchens fairfieldfarmkitchens.com
NATURE'S ORGANIC	**Nature's Organic Goodness** Barrie, ONT L4N 8Z6 800-353-3178	**ORGANIC GOURMET**	**Organic Gourmet** Sherman Oaks, CA 91403 800-400-7772 organic-gourmet.com
NATURE'S PATH	**Nature's Path** Vancouver, BC 888-808-9505 Family owned naturespath.com	**ORGANIC PLANET**	**Organic Planet** Philadelphia, PA 19119 215-753-7171 organicplanet.com
NEWMAN'S OWN	**Newman's Own** Westport, CT 06880 516-625-2600 Family owned newmansown.com	**Our Family Farm**	**Our Family Farm** Newport, KY 41071 859-261-2627 Family owned ourfamilyfarm.com
	Nielsen-Massey Waukegan, IL 60085 800-525-7873 Family owned nielsenmassey.com	**Pamela's**	**Pamela's Products** San Francisco, CA 650-952-4546 pamelasproducts.com

AISLE 7 GUIDE TO BRANDS

Company Logo	Contact/Corporate Information	Company Logo	Contact/Corporate Information
Pastorelli	**Pastorelli** Chicago, IL 60607 800-767-2829 pastorelli.com	**Raised Right**	**Raised Right** Fredericksburg, PA 17026 717-865-2136 College Hill Poultry Kreamer Feed raisedright.com
	Paul's Grains Laurel, IA 50141 641-476-3373 Family owned paulsgrains.com	**Rapunzel** true to nature	**Rapunzel** Valatie, NY 12184 800-207-2814 rapunzel.com
PEACE CEREAL	**Peace Cereal** Eugene, OR 800-225-3623 Golden Temple peacecereal.com	**Rigoni USA** ORGANIC FARMING	**Rigoni Organic** Oxford, CT 06478 203-267-3280 Rigoni USA rigoniusa.com
PERRICONE	**Perricone Juices, Inc.** Beaumont, CA 92223 909-769-7171 Family owned perriconejuices.com	**RISING MOON ORGANICS**	**Rising Moon Organics** Eugene, OR 97402 541-431-0505 risingmoon.com
PETALUMA POULTRY	**Petaluma Poultry** Petaluma, CA 94955 707-763-1904 petalumapoultry.com	**Road's End Organics**	**Road's End Organics** Morrisville, VT 05661 877-CHREESE chreese.com
PINE CREEK PACK NATURAL	**Pine Creek Pack** Omak, WA 98841 509-826-8003 Fruit grower coalition pinecreekpack.com		**Rocamojo, Inc.** Woodland Hills, CA 91367 818-961-0485 rocamojo.com
Pure Luck Texas	**Pure Luck Texas** Dripping Springs, TX 78620 512-858-7034 Independently owned purelucktexas.com		**Rock Spring Farm** Spring Grove, MN 55974 563-735-5613 rsfarm.com Ⓡ
purity. Organic	**Purity Organic Juices** Watsonville, CA 415-673-5555 purityorganic.com	**Rudi's** ORGANIC	**Rudi's** Boulder, CO 80301 877-293-0876 Rudi's Organic Bakery rudisbakery.com

AISLE 7 GUIDE TO BRANDS

Company Logo	Contact/Corporate Information	Company Logo	Contact/Corporate Information
RYVITA	**Ryvita** Paramus, NJ 07652 201-909-0808 InterNatural Foods internaturalfoods.com	Small Planet Foods	**Small Planet Foods** Sedro-Woolley, WA 98284 800-624-4123 General Mills cfarm.com
Seabreeze Organic Farm	**Seabreeze Organic Farm** San Diego, CA 92130 858-481-0209 Family owned CSA seabreezed.com	**SMOKE & FIRE** *Soy with Sizzle*	**Smoke & Fire Natural Foods** Great Barrington, MA 01230 413-528-6891 smokeandfire.com
Seapoint Farms	**Seapoint Farms** Huntington Beach, CA 92648 714-841-9831 seapointfarms.com	Sno-Pac	**Sno-Pac** Caledonia, MN 55921 800-533-2215 Family owned snopac.com
Season's	**Season's** Addison, IL 60101 630-628-0211 seasonssnacks.com	**SO NICE ORGANIC**	**So Nice Soyganic** Vancouver, BC V6B 3X5 888-401-0019 Soyaworld, Inc. sonice-soyganic.com
SEEDS OF CHANGE	**Seeds of Change** Vernon, CA 90058 888-762-4240 M&M Mars seedsofchange.com	So Soya+	**So Soya** Markham, ONT L3R 2M9 905-948-1769 sosoyaplus.com
seven cups	**Seven Cups Teas** Tucson, AZ 85754 866-997-2877 Green Dragon Enterprises sevencups.com		**Solana Gold Organics** Sebastopol, CA 95473 800-459-1121 solanagold.com
ShariAnn's ORGANIC	**ShariAnn's Organic** Garden City, NY 11530 800-434-4246 Hain-Celestial / Heinz shariannsorganic.com	SONORA MILLS	**Sonora Mills Foods** Rancho Dominguez, CA 90221 310-639-5333 sonoramills.com
SIMPLY ORGANIC	**Simply Organic** Norway, IA 52318 800-729-5422 Frontier National Brands (co-op) frontierherb.com	SOUTH TEX ORGANICS	**South Tex Organics** Mission, TX 78572 888-895-0108 Family owned stxorganics.com

AISLE 7 GUIDE TO BRANDS

Company Logo	Contact/Corporate Information	Company Logo	Contact/Corporate Information
	Southern Brown Rice Weiner, AR 72479 800-421-7423 southernbrownrice.com	SUNSPIRE Candies	**Sunspire** San Leandro, CA 94577 510-569-9731 nSpired Natural Foods sunspire.com
	Soy Deli S. San Francisco, CA 94080 650-553-9900 Quong Hop & Co. quonghop.com		**Sweet Cactus Farms** Los Angeles, CA 90232 310-733-4343 sweetcactusfarms.com
Turtle Mountain	**Soy Delicious** Eugene, OR 21938 541-338-9400 Turtle Mountain turtlemountain.com		**Sweet Grass Farms** Kalispell, MT 59901 406-755-3711 sweetgrassfarms.com
SOY DREAM	**Soy Dream** Garden City, NY 11530 800-333-6339 Imagine Foods Hain-Celestial/Heinz imaginefoods.com	SWEET ORGANICS	**Sweet Organics** Addison, IL 60101 630-628-0211 Kettle Cooked Chips Season's Enterprises seasonssnacks.com
SOY FUSION	**Soy Fusion** Saline, MI 313-429-2310 American Soy Products americansoy.com	Tartex	**Tartex** Acton, ONT L7J 2L7 519-853-3899 Anke Kruse Organics ankekruseorganics.com
SOYCO FOODS	**Soyco** Orlando, FL 32809 800-855-5500 Galaxy Foods galaxyfoods.com	TERRA	**Terra Chips** Melville, NY 11747 631-730-2200 Hain-Celestial Heinz terrachips.com
Spectrum Naturals Organic	**Spectrum Organic Products, Inc.** Petaluma, CA 94954 800-995-2705 spectrumorganics.com	TERRA NOSTRA organic	**Terra Nostra Organic** Vancouver, BC V6N 4J9 604-267-3582 KFM Foods International terranostra.us
SUNRIDGE FARMS	**SunRidge Farms** Santa Cruz, CA 95062 831-462-1280 sunridgefarms.com		**Thanksgiving Coffee Co.** Fort Bragg, CA 95437 800-648-6491 thanksgivingcoffee.com

AISLE 7 GUIDE TO BRANDS

Company Logo	Contact/Corporate Information	Company Logo	Contact/Corporate Information
Tiensvold Farms	**Tiensvold Farms** Rushville, NE 69360 308-327-3135 eatorganicbuffalo.com	Walnut Acres Organic	**Walnut Acres** New Rochelle, NY 10801 800-222-3276 Hain-Celestial Heinz walnutacres.com
Tierra Vegetables	**Tierra Vegetables** Healdsburg, CA 95448 888-7TIERRA tierravegetables.com	Waymouth Farms	**Waymouth Farms Organic** New Hope, MN 55428 763-533-5300 Waymouth Farms, Inc. goodsensesnacks.com
Traditional Medicinals	**Traditional Medicinals** Sebastopol, CA 95472 800-543-4372 traditionalmedicinals.com	Westbrae Natural	**Westbrae Natural** Garden City, NY 11530 800-434-4246 Hain-Celestial Heinz westbrae.com
Traverse Bay Farms The Art of Healthy Eating	**Traverse Bay Farms** Bellaire, MI 49615 877-746-7477 traversebayfarms.com	Wholesome Sweeteners	**Wholesome Sweeteners** Sugarland, TX 77478 281-490-3582 Imperial Sugar Company wholesomesweeteners.com
Up Country Organics	**Up Country Organics** St. Johnsbury, VT 05819 802-748-5141 upcountryorganics.com	wisdom	**Wisdom Herbs** Bonduel, WI 54107 800-899-9908 wisdomherbs.com
ViVANi Premium Organic	**Vivani** Paramus, NJ 07652 201-909-0808 InterNatural Foods internaturalfoods.com	Wizard's	**Wizard's Cauldron** Yanceyville, NC 27379 336-694-5665 Edward & Sons Trading Co. wizardscauldron.com
Walkers	**Walkers** Hauppauge, NY 11788 631-273-0011 walkersshortbread.com		

CONCLUSION
Beyond the Checkout Counter

IN THE LAST TEN YEARS, government oversight, corporate involvement, and increased media attention have moved organics from the food-buying fringes onto mainstream supermarket shelves. From produce to packaged goods, you now confront a dizzying variety of new products and brand names. As even more items become available, the question that sparked our journey of discovery remains: *Is organic food worth it?*

The volume of information on the subject is staggering and often confusing. Organic advocates cite a long list of reasons to condemn conventional agriculture and buy organic. Critics of organic food charge that it represents nothing more than a corporate cash cow based on questionable science and fear-based marketing.

So here we are at the end of more than two years of research and writing. Along the way we have read and heard the words of supporters, detractors, farmers, government officials, friends, family, and even those with little or no interest in the subject. All have contributed valuable insights as we—setting aside our preconceived notions—shaped our ideas.

For the record, here are our own opinions and conclusions, organized by issue.

HEALTH

Although we are sympathetic to consumers' and producers' concerns about food-related health issues, we believe many of these issues have been exaggerated. While health fears attract attention, organic advocates could better serve both the movement and the industry if they used fears as springboards to furthering knowledge, rather than allowing them to become the sole focus of market researchers and consumers alike. Nevertheless, when it comes to health issues, we offer these few conclusions:

There is little or no substantial difference in nutrient content, bacterial contamination, and appearance between organic and conventional food.

Organic foods contain fewer currently used pesticide residues.

- Residues are routinely found on many produce items—including organic, although to a lesser degree. These amounts are very small and rarely exceed the levels deemed safe by the FDA. Many of the residues found are from long-banned pesticides that are still in the environment, and organic food is not immune to this kind of contamination. While pesticide residues may affect health, definitive studies have not, as yet, proven that they do.
- There is much discussion regarding children's increased susceptibility to pesticides. The Food Quality Protection Act of 1996 put several new safeguards in place to protect children. But testing on older yet still currently registered pesticides is not yet complete, so caution is

warranted. Still, evidence of widespread problems from *residue contamination* is still scarce. Of more concern than residues in food are the health effects on children resulting from household pesticides. We believe that if your budget allows, it makes sense to buy organic foods eaten often by your children; but do not be fearful of allowing children to eat conventional produce. The health effects of not eating any fresh produce still outweigh the potential for problems.

Buying organic dairy products may not be worth the extra cost, unless you live in a state with large dairy factories.

- Except for butter, conventional dairy products seldom contain pesticide residues other than DDT, which can also be found in organic dairy products.
- Antibiotic residues are not allowed in any milk.
- IGF-1 is a natural component of milk. The amount present in milk fluctuates depending on the cycle of the cow, and it cannot be determined whether rBST has been used.
- Large factory-type dairies present more problems across the board. They are found primarily now in California and Arizona, although they are slowly beginning to emerge in other states, such as Florida, Colorado, and Idaho. Nationally branded organic dairy products may come from very large herds.

Organic meat is somewhat safer than conventional meat.

- The use of antibiotics in cattle is waning, and their residues are not allowed in beef, but evidence shows that antibiotic abuse leads to resistant strains of bacteria.
- It is highly unlikely that BSE will be found in any organic beef. On the same account, BSE has not become a major problem for conventional U.S. beef, but critics charge that

adequate safeguards to prevent mad cow have not yet been fully implemented.

- Hormones in conventional beef are measured in nanograms, and there is no indication that these small amounts are a health problem for most adults. The jury is still out in whether they are a problem for small children and pregnant women.
- Growth hormones are not allowed in either conventional or organic chickens or hogs.
- Organic chickens have not been fed antibiotics.

THE ENVIRONMENT

When it comes to the environment, organic principles offer some clear advantages. Reducing agriculture's dependence on synthetic chemicals has been, is now, and forever will be a good idea. But conventional agriculture doesn't use these chemicals *solely* for the purpose of lining the pockets of large chemical corporations. Pesticides and synthetic chemicals were developed for specific reasons. Obviously these technologies could be improved or discontinued in the future, but there's a world to feed out there. Will a larger demand for organic food solve the environmental problems caused by conventional farming in the United States? No, at least not now, but agriculture *does* negatively impact the environment, and the practice of organic farming *is—in most cases— more environmentally sound*. Here are our findings:

Organic farming practices can help control ground- and surface-water contamination.

Small organic farms encourage biodiversity more than conventional farms.

Less than one percent of all U.S. cropland is certified organic, making the beneficial effects small and localized.

- Nearly half of all certified acres are range and pasture land, not cropland.
- We are not yet close to having the needed quantity of organic acreage to have large-scale impact on the environment, but buying from your small local producers could have a direct effect on your own neck of the woods.

Time is running out.

- The number of acres transitioning to organic is not rising quickly enough to meet the demand.
- Cheaper organic imports have begun to fill the void, but hope remains for the future of better agricultural practices. Colleges and universities offer courses in organic farming, and a new generation seems poised to take up the causes and practices of the early organic practitioners.

Organic farms are getting larger.

- Most of the increased organic acreages are not happening on small, quaint farms but rather on large, industrial organic farms. Average size increased from 140 acres in 1997 to 185 acres in 2002.[1] This growth parallels conventional agriculture's drive toward ever-greater efficiency. Despite organic methods, large farms will always present more environmental problems than smaller, more intensely managed ones.
- Many large organic distributors *currently* pool products from small farms. As in the conventional system, smaller producers eventually get squeezed out in favor of larger, more efficient farms.

Although it still requires vigilance, erosion may not be the crisis it is made out to be.

- In the past twenty years U.S. farmers have cut the amount of erosion by more than a third.
- If erosion were a crisis, U.S. farm yields would be falling. They are not.

Over time organic standards will probably weaken and allow more destructive practices.

- As more organic foods are shifted into the mainstream, the industry will seek a scale of efficiency that the current standards impede. Several attempts have already been made to weaken the standards. So far these attempts have been public enough to elicit widespread condemnation. The history of the food industry is rife with rule-bending, back-patting, and outright deceptions that weaken regulations over time, and the NOP rule will be no exception.

SOCIETY

Perhaps the most positive, endearing, and idealistic aspect of the organic movement is its social values. Although the organic principles of fair trade and economic justice, better treatment of labor, localized food systems, and equitable food distribution have not been completely realized, the organic movement has sparked debate about them. More people, especially young people, are now aware of the many problems facing the future of agriculture.

- The amount of land dedicated to organic research more than doubled between 2001 and 2003, although most of the funding came from corporate, not public, interests.

- Organic agriculture's higher prices have helped some farmers, but the organic industry views price premiums as an obstacle to market expansion, leading to economies of scale similar to those in conventional production.
- We predict that this trend will result in some kind of synthesis of conventional and organic farming practices. Although this synthesis will water down organic standards, a small positive effect on the agricultural system as a whole will result. But it will not necessarily build the system (or the soil) in the way the organic pioneers envisioned.
- Even though large multinational corporations express little interest in social concerns, their entrance into the organic arena has changed the way they do business. This is a good thing, although it tends to make organic a profit center rather than a way of life. In the words of John Mellencamp, "Ain't that America."

FINAL THOUGHTS

The original plan for Dan to play devil to Luddene's organic advocacy didn't exactly work out. While operating an organic market garden on an acre of a conventional dairy farm, she started questioning some of the information she encountered about conventional dairies and began to doubt some of the claims organic advocates were making. He, on the other hand, spent his days in grain elevators battling pests, awestruck by the massive amounts of food that industrial agriculture produces, and questioning his small role in the system.

But Luddene's skepticism did not cloud her vision about the very real, perennial problems with agriculture or her belief in traditional organic principles. Nor did Dan's musings about finding a better way result in a complete road-to-Damascus-like conversion. (He did, however, join his local co-op, cut down meat consumption, and whenever possible, buys produce from always-friendly local farmers at roadside stands and farmers markets.)

The result has been a meeting of minds, and a recognition that organic agriculture is worth it in the sense that it plays a vital role as a vehicle for change. With its long history of passionate and steadfast belief, and a growing role in the marketplace of ideas, organics can and should function as a tool to reshape our understanding of what it means to grow food and of the importance of doing so in more sustainable ways.

Which brings us back to our original question: *Is organic food worth it?* The answer *cannot* be a simple yes or no, despite all the articles, books, and websites telling you what to think and which foods to buy. The answer can only be found in the interaction between you and the knowledge you seek. We have attempted to provide you with a broader and deeper understanding about what is at stake in the organic agriculture debate—an internal debate that you engage in every time you stand in a supermarket aisle examining a piece of fruit and calculating the added cost.

Is eating organic foods a healthier option? Will buying organic foods halt global warming? Will your purchase of organic food change the world? In the end, only you can decide.

Shop well.

Notes

Chapter 1: Organics 101

1. U.S. citizens pay, on average, about 7.1 percent of their earnings for food. Compared to the British (who pay about 10 percent), and the Indians (who pay about 48 percent), Americans have it good.

2. We originally included 1890 figures—43 percent of the workforce—from the Economic Research Service of the USDA, on their website at www.usda.gov/history2/text3.htm, but it appears this fine history of agriculture resource has either been removed or has been closed for renovations. In its place, we have used the figure cited by former Secretary of Agriculture Dan Glickman: "In 1900, farmers represented 38 percent of the labor force. By 1950, the number of farms had decreased only by a few hundred thousand, but farmers dropped to only 12 percent of the labor force. By 1990, there were barely 2 million farms, and farmers made up 2.6 percent of the workforce. Sixty years of aggressive farm programs have not been able to reverse this trend." Dan Glickman (remarks, Purdue University, West Lafayette, IN, April 29, 1999), www.biotech-info.net/purdue glickman.html.

3. Randy Lloyd, "The Ag School Room." University of Illinois, www. urbanext.uiuc.edu/mclean/school/school

room0212.html. In 2001, only 1.8 percent of the American population engaged in farming, which means that more Americans are incarcerated than working the farms.

4. Robert N. Anderson, "United States Life Tables, 1997," *National Vital Statistics Reports* 47, no. 28 (December 13, 1999). Table 11, "Life Expectancy by Age, Race and Sex," for selected years 1929–98, www.cdc.gov/nchs/data/nvsr/nvsr47/nvs47_28.pdf. In 1900, life expectancy was 47.88 years for white males and 50.70 for white females. In 1997 it was 73.6 for white males and 79.4 for white females. The average is 27.21 years longer.

5. When organic food became a bona fide industry in need of regulation, different ideas about what *organic* really meant created confusion. Definitions and standards varied; so did causes and concerns. Different states and organizations had different production rules about labeling standards, which in turn led to turf wars and ideological impasses. In the eyes of many within the fledgling organic industry, government involvement seemed like a solution. After years of discussion and the adoption of government standards, many small organic farmers and advocates now can be heard muttering, "Be careful what you wish for," in the halls of conferences and trade shows.

6. Exact statistics are a little confusing. While the NOP cites ninety-four agencies, a quick count reveals ninety-six. Other sources have quoted figures from 120 to 137. See www.ams.usda.gov/nop/CertifyingAgents/AccreditationStatus.html.

7. "Product Composition ... (b) Products sold, labeled, or represented as 'organic' must contain (by weight or fluid volume, excluding water and salt) not less than 95 percent organically produced raw or processed agricultural products. Any remaining product ingredients

must be organically produced, unless not commercially available in organic form." *CFR,* vol. 65 §205.301 (2000) 80646.

8. *CFR,* National Organic Program Overview, Subpart D "Labeling Products 'Made With Organic (specified ingredients or food group[s]),' " 80579.

Chapter 2: The Evolution of Organic Agriculture

1. Harvey Levenstein, *Revolution at the Table* (Berkeley: University of California Press, 2003), and *Paradox of Plenty* (London: Oxford University Press, 2003).

2. J. I. Rodale, "Why I Started Organic Gardening," *The Best of Organic Gardening* (Emmaus, PA: Rodale Press, 1996), 7.

3. Sir Albert Howard, "How to Avoid a Famine of Quality," *Organic Gardening,* November 1947.

4. State of Pennsylvania Department of Environmental Protection, "J. I. Rodale and the Rodale Family Celebrating 50 Years as Advocates for Sustainable Agriculture," www.dep.state.pa.us/dep/PA_Env-Her/rodale_bio.htm.

5. Rodale, "Why I Started Organic Gardening," 8.

6. Donald W. Lotter, "Organic Agriculture," *Journal of Sustainable Agriculture* 21, no. 4 (2003). Perhaps Rodale was inspired by Lord Northburne's 1940 book *Look to the Land.*

7. Rodale, "Why I Started Organic Gardening," 4.

Chapter 3: Organic Foods and Your Health

1. Survey by the Hartman Group as reported in *Organic Business News,* March 2001.

2. Michael Pollan, "Behind the Organic Industrial Complex," *New York Times Magazine*, May 13, 2001.
3. May R. Berenbaum, *Bugs in the System: Insects and Their Impact on Human Affairs* (Reading, MA: Helix Books, 1995), 284.
4. Pest-control technology is constantly improving. The concern about chemicals in the environment has led to a number of new approaches to the problem. The old paradigm of pest eradication has given way to more ecologically based ideas, such as biopesticides, and integrated pest management strategies. In addition, organic and other forms of "eco-friendly" agriculture point to the basic problem of monocultures, insisting that a more diverse agricultural environment naturally reduces the pests that accompany large fields of the same crop. The challenge for the future of pest control is to develop agricultural systems that are less vulnerable to pests but still produce high yields.
5. This table shows pesticide use in the United States for 1999 (in millions of pounds):

Type of Pesticide	Agriculture Use	Commercial Use	Home Use	Total	Allowed in Organics
Herbicides	470	48	49	567	0
Fumigants	140	24	1	165	0
Insecticides	184	30	17	231	102
Fungicides	131	20	8	159	78
Growth Regulators	165	N/A	N/A	N/A	75
Total in 1999	1,090	122	75	1,287	255

6. H. Patricia Hynes, *Earthright*. (Rocklin, CA: Prima, 1990), 18.
7. Organic Materials Review Institute, "Generic Materials

List" (Eugene, OR: Organic Materials Review Institute, 2002).

8. USDA, Economic Research Service, "Organic Production," (2002), tables 5 and 6, www.ers.usda.gov/data/organic.

9. FDA, Center for Food Safety and Applied Nutrition, "Pesticide Program, Residue Monitoring, 2002," www.cfsan.fda.gov/~dms/pes02rep.html#tdsresults. The table below from the CFSAN report lists the twenty most *frequently* found residues (in descending order) and the range of amounts in the four market baskets analyzed in 2002 (1,030 food items). The levels of these residues are well below regulatory limits.

Pesticide	Range, ppm	Pesticide	Range, ppm
DDT*	0.0001–0.025	thiabendazole	0.013–0.991
chlorpyrifos-methyl	0.0002–0.059	lindane*	0.0001–0.002
malathion	0.0007–0.071	methamidophos	0.001–0.345
Endosulfan	0.0001–0.166	hexachlorobenzene*	0.0001–0.002
dieldrin*	0.0001–0.010	dicofol	0.002–0.538
chlorpropham	0.0007–1.278	pirimiphos-methyl	0.001–0.024
chlorpyrifos	0.0001–0.105	quintozene	0.0001–0.0424
permethrin	0.0004–1.680	toxaphene*	0.002–0.028
carbaryl	0.001–2.040	acephate	0.002–0.350
dicloran	0.0002–0.263	ethion	0.0003–0.007

* Banned or highly restricted

10. Ruth A. Etzel, Sophie J. Balk, eds., *Pediatric Environmental Health,* 2nd ed. (Elk Grove Village, IL: American Academy of Pediatrics, 2004), 169.

11. Ibid, 341.

12. Rebecca Renner, "Nietzche's Toxicology," *Scientific American,* August 2003. A recent *Scientific American*

article discusses a growing body of research that suggests low-level exposures to environmental contaminants may not actually be poisonous but rather strength-building. Called *hormesis,* "this phenomenon appears to be an adaptive response to stress." Study of this phenomenon is in its infancy, but it is "raising more questions than answers" about the long-held "dose-makes-the-poison" assumptions of modern toxicology.

13. "Organic. It's Lower in Pesticides. Honest," *Consumer Reports,* August 2002. The findings of this report, published in *Food Additives and Contaminants,* confirm that organic produce does indeed minimize the risk to pesticide residue exposure, although it does not guarantee pesticide-free food. In addition, the report points out the fact that pesticides allowed in organic production are not tested for at all. According to the summary, "there is no objective evidence to support the assertion that natural pesticide residues pose a hazard." The same could be said for synthetic pesticide residues.

14. *CFR,* vol. 65, §205.238, 80645.

15. There were approximately one million organic chickens in 2001, compared with 9.3 billion conventional ones. This equates to 15,625 pounds of antibiotics not being used in organics, compared to 29.5 million pounds used in conventional agriculture.

16. Maverick Beef Ranch, www.maverickranch.com/ health_and_nutrition/beef_facts_myths.cfm.

17. In the 1960s and 1970s, the FDA canceled the use of many food additives, particularly artificial colors. Anxiety over additives was directed toward cancer, birth defects, and allergic reactions, plus various other minor ailments. The flavor enhancer monosodium glutamate (MSG) made headlines for several years as being the cause for "Chinese Restaurant Syndrome"—the headaches, dizziness, and chest pains some people

experience after dining on Chinese food. With the accompanying media attention, consumers began to read labels. Natural food advocate Beatrice Trum Hunter summed up the public's concerns as far back as 1961: "From the consumer's viewpoint, most of these additives are unnecessary. They have no nutritive value. They are used by the food industry for economic advantage in a highly competitive market. Foods treated in this manner may appear brighter and may last longer, but the people who eat them don't." Beatrice Trum Hunter, *The Natural Foods Cookbook* (New York: Simon & Schuster, 1961), 11. The FDA quelled the storm by banning some additives.

18. Because humans have been genetically *modifying* living things (dogs, sheep, pigs, petunias, racehorses, apples, corn, etc.) for centuries, we have chosen to refer to the new techniques as genetic *engineering* instead of genetic *modification*. Despite what some antibiotechnology activists say, cross-breeding plants the old-fashioned way *is* a modification. Acknowledging this fact preempts the counterargument offered by biotech researchers that we have always genetically modified plants and that biotechnology changes nothing. It *does* change something.

19. Human insulin for diabetics was the first successful product developed using this method. Critics of GEOs cite several problems with this insulin, but proponents claim it has saved millions of diabetics' lives by increasing the availability and significantly lowering its price.

20. Thomas R. DeGregori, *Origins of the Organic Agriculture Debate* (Ames: Iowa State Press, 2004), 83.

21. Fertilizer labels are required to list the percentage of nutrients. Usually these are listed as NPK, the chemical letters representing the elements nitrogen, phosphorus, and potassium. A number on a fertilizer label,

such as 10-15-10 means that for every hundred pounds, the fertilizer supplies ten pounds of nitrogen, fifteen pounds of phosphorus, and ten pounds of potassium.

22. Virginia Worthington, "Nutritional Quality of Organic Versus Conventional Fruits, Vegetables, and Grains," *Journal of Alternative and Complementary Medicine* 7, no. 2 (2001): 161–73.

23. Thomas R. DeGregori, *Bountiful Harvest: Technology, Food Safety, and The Environment* (Washington: CATO Institute, 2002), 97.

24. P. T. Tybor, and Warren Gilson, "Dairy Producer's Guide to Food Safety in Milk Production." University of Georgia College of Agriculture and Environmental Science, http://pubscaes.uga.edu/caespubs/pubcd/B1084-W.HTML.

25. Niels Maness, "Peanut," in *The Commercial Storage of Fruits, Vegetables, and Florist and Nursery Stocks, Agriculture Handbook Number 66* (Washington: USDA, 2004), www.ba.ars.usda.gov/hb66/160peanut.pdf.

Chapter 4: Organic Foods and the Environment

1. Michael Pollan, "Behind the Organic Industrial Complex," *New York Times Magazine,* May 13, 2001.

2. A possible exception is the work being done at The Land Institute in Salina, Kansas. There, Wes Jackson has been experimenting with farming systems that make use of perennials in a carefully constructed polyculture that if successful will, "like a prairie, [run] entirely on sunlight and rain." Scott Russel Sanders, "Learning from the Prairie," in *The New Agrarianism,* ed. Eric T. Freyfogle (Washington: Island Press, 2001), 5.

3. Erosion is difficult to accurately measure and is often

a localized problem (such as a hillside). Therefore broad trends cannot account for some of these problems (see accompanying graph).

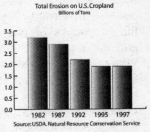

Total Erosion on U.S. Cropland
Billions of Tons

Source: USDA, Natural Resource Conservation Service

4. David Norse, "Fertilizers and Food Demand: Implications for Environmental Stresses," *Agro-Chemical Report* 3, no. 2 (April–June 2003), www.fadinap.org/nib/nib2003_2/aprjun03-4-focus.pdf.

5. Ibid.

6. Corn, soybeans, wheat, and rice are the most frequently planted crops in the United States and account for over 52 percent of the 450 million acres of cropland.

Chapter 5: Organic Foods and Society

1. Eliot Coleman, "Beyond Organic," *Mother Earth News* (December– January 2002), 89.

2. R. Douglas Hurt, *Problems of Plenty* (Chicago: Ivan P. Dee, 2002). Some would argue that the whole farm crisis is based on the point that the farmer cannot set his or her own prices.

3. Earthbound Farms, www.ebfarm.com/About/EarthboundStory.aspx.

4. The organic method can be accomplished in a closed system without purchased off-farm inputs, but doing so is extremely difficult and time consuming. Organic farmers have developed a number of "approved" nutrient sources that manufacturers are only too happy to produce. These include: humates, alfalfa meal, kelp

products, various liquid, powdered, and pelletized fish products, bat guano, blood meal, bone meal, corn gluten, ground crab shells, feather meal, compost teas, greensand, gypsum powder, neemcake, soybean meal, worm castings, mined minerals, oyster shells, oat bran, molasses, and shrimp shells. All these products are highly processed and are transported considerable distances. One popular supplier of organic nutrients provides nearly a hundred products, many in fifty-pound bags. They conveniently include commercial trucking rates for large orders.

5. See the National Center for Farmworker Health website, www. ncfh.org/docs/fs-Occ%20Health.pdf.

6. "These phrases may be consumer friendly but clearly do not convey the extensive and complex nature of contemporary organic agriculture. These phrases may be used as additional eco-labels, provided they are truthful labeling statements. They are not permitted as replacements for the term 'organic'." *CFR*, Uses of Other Terms as Synonymous for "Organic" (7), 80586.

7. Bill Liebhardt, "Get the Facts Straight: Organic Yields Are Good," *Organic Farming Research Foundation Information Bulletin,* no. 10 (Summer 2001), 4.

8. Paul R. Mahoney, "Profitability of Organic Cropping Systems in Southwestern Minnesota," www.misa.umn. edu/Other/profitabilityorganiccropping.html, 13.

Part II: Navigating the Aisles

1. These statistics come from the USDA's National Agricultural Statistics Service found at www.usda.gov/ nass/. The USDA maintains thousands of statistics regarding many aspects of production, such as chemicals used, manure used, crop rotations, amounts produced, and so on. While it keeps some for organic production,

the extent of the data is limited. In all cases, we have used the latest year available at time of writing.

2. USDA, Economic Research Service, "U.S. Farming, 2000–2001," www.usda.gov/data/Organic. These statistics are not maintained yearly, and release dates are sporadic.

Aisle 1: The Produce Department

1. "The Earthbound Farm Story," www.ebfarm.com/About/EarthboundStory.aspx.

2. Christine Blank, "Organic Poultry and Egg Production Increases as Sales Heat Up," *Organic Business News* 16, no. 7 (2004), 6.

3. Catherine Green, "Recent Growth Patterns in the U.S. Organic Food Market," Economic Research Service, USDA, (2000), 11.

4. "Organic. It's Lower in Pesticides. Honest," *Consumer Reports,* August 2002, citing *Journal of Food Additives and Contaminants* 19, no. 5 (2002), www.consumerreports.org.

5. Charles Benbrook, "Minimizing Pesticide Dietary Exposure Through the Consumption of Organic Food," Organic Center for Education and Promotion (2004), www.organiccenter.org/science.htm?groupid=4&articleid=25, 9.

6. The Grimm brothers, Rod and Bob (it's a family farm!), process nine million carrots per day and package them under thirty different labels. Grimmway Farms and its main competitor, Bolthouse Farms, control 80 percent of the California carrot industry. See www.grimmway.com/about_history_californian.html.

7. Michelle Le Strange, Wayne L. Schrader, Timothy K. Hartz, "Fresh-Market Tomato Production in California," University of California, Vegetable Research and

Information Center, Publication no. 8017, http://anrcatalog.ucdavis.edu/pdf/8017.pdf.

8. Steve Diver, George Kuepper, and Holly Born, "Organic Tomato Production," National Sustainable Agriculture Information Service (March 1999), http://attra.ncat.org/attra-pub/tomato.html#appendices.

9. D. N. Maynard et al. "Tomato Production in Florida—HS739," University of Florida, IFAS Extension (September 2003), http://edis.ifas.ufl.edu/pdffiles/CV/CV13700.pdf.

10. "Pesticide Use Database," National Center for Food and Agriculture Policy, www.ncfap.org/pesticidedb.htm.

11. Diver, Kuepper, and Born, "Organic Tomato Production."

12. Andrew Kimbrell, *The Fatal Harvest Reader* (Washington: Island Press, 2002), 182.

13. Michael Colt, Ronda Hirnyck, Tom Lyon, "Crop Profile for Apples in Idaho (Tree Nutrition)," University of Idaho (June 2001), http://pestdata.ncsu.edu/cropprofiles/docs/Idapples.html.

14. Guy K. Ames and George Kuepper, "Overview of Organic Fruit Production," Appropriate Technology Transfer for Rural Areas (February 2000), http://attra.ncat.org/attra-pub/PDF/fruitover.pdf, 8.

Aisle 2: Breads, Cereals, Pasta, and Grains

1. R. Douglas Hurt, *Problems of Plenty* (Chicago: Ivan P. Dee, 2002), 12.

2. *Yearbook of the United States Department of Agriculture: 1919* (Washington: USDA), 19.

3. George Frisvold, John Sullivan, and Anton Raneses, "Who gains from genetic improvements in US crops?"

AgBioForum, 2(3&4) (1999), www.agbioforum.org/v2n34/v2n34a15-frisvold.htm, 237–46.

4. Lynda Brown, *The Shopper's Guide to Organic Food* (London: Fourth Estate, 1998), 225.

5. *CFR,* vol. 65 (2000), §205.203(e) (3), 80644.

6. Andrew Kimbrell, "A Blow to the Breadbasket: Industrial Grain Production," *The Fatal Harvest Reader,* 101.

7. USDA, National Resources Conservation Service, "National Resources Inventory" (2000), www.nrcs.usda.gov/technical/land/lgif/m5848l.gif.

8. To meet future needs of organic products, here is a look at what must happen. Industry sales figures are from *Progressive Grocer* magazine and are from 2002 with the standard 1 percent increase added to the subsequent figures. The organic sales figures are from the OTA's website. Projections for organic sales are based on a 20 percent increase.

The Future of Organics?

Year	U.S. Grocery industry revenue at 1% growth rate	Organic Production Revenue	% of U.S. Total Food $	Total Needed Certified Organic Acres	% of U.S. Total Acres	Annual Increase in Organic Acres	Number of New Organic Farms Needed	% of Total U.S. Farms
2003	540,754,000,000	10,380,000,000	1.92	2,343,924	0.28		9,567	0.45
2004	546,161,540,000	12,456,000,000	2.28	2,812,709	0.34	468,785	1,913	0.54
2005	551,623,155,400	14,947,200,000	2.71	3,375,251	0.41	562,542	2,296	0.65
2006	557,139,386,954	17,936,640,000	3.22	4,050,301	0.49	675,050	2,755	0.78
2007	562,710,780,824	21,523,968,000	3.83	4,860,361	0.59	810,060	3,306	0.93
2008	568,337,888,632	25,828,761,600	4.54	5,832,433	0.70	972,072	3,968	1.12
2009	574,021,267,518	30,994,513,920	5.40	6,998,920	0.85	1,166,487	4,761	1.34
2010	579,761,480,193	37,193,416,704	6.42	8,398,703	1.01	1,399,784	5,713	1.61
2011	585,559,094,995	44,632,100,045	7.62	10,078,444	1.22	1,679,741	6,856	1.93
2012	591,414,685,945	53,558,520,054	9.06	12,094,133	1.46	2,015,689	8,227	2.32

Total New Organic Farmers Needed by 2012: 39,797

Aisle 3: Seeds, Beans, Nuts, and Oils

1. Judith Putnam and Jane E. Allshouse, "Food Consumption, Prices, and Expenditures, 1970–97," Economic Research Service, *Statistical Bulletin,* no. 965 (Washington: USDA, 1999), 21.

2. Ibid, 74.

3. "Fun Tidbits," Jif Peanut Butter, www.jif.com/aboutjif/aj_tidbits.asp.

4. National Organic Standard Board. *Final Recommendation Addendum Number 12: Allowable Methods of Oil Extraction for Processed Foods* (October 31, 1995).

5. "Trans fatty acids increase LDL cholesterol and reduce HDL cholesterol levels. On a gram for gram basis, *trans* fats have approximately twice the adverse effect of saturated fatty acids on the LDL/HDL ratio, which is a strong predictor of coronary heart disease. Furthermore, *trans* fats increase triglyceride levels compared to saturated fats. Also, in prospective epidemiological studies, *trans* fats have strongly predicted risk of future coronary heart disease. Omega-3 fatty acids, found in some vegetable sources, inhibit platelet aggregation at high intakes and have been hypothesized to reduce risk of coronary heart disease." Walter Willett, M.D., "Trans and Omega-3 Fatty Acids and CUD Risk," paper presented at "Diet and Optimum Health" conference, Linus Pauling Institute, Corvallis, Oregon, May 2001, http://lpi.oregonstate.edu/conference/willett1.html.

6. FDA, Center for Food Safety and Applied Nutrition, "Pesticide Program, Residue Monitoring, 2002," www.cfsan.fda.gov/~dms/pes02rep.html#tdsresults.

7. From the package of Newman's Own Chocolate Crème-Filled Cookies.

8. Fred Rohe, *Eat Fat—Your Life Depends on It* (Middletown, CA: Organic Marketing, 2000), 20.

Aisle 4: The Dairy Case

1. Marilyn Nestle, *Food Politics* (Berkeley: University of California Press, 2002), 79. More than eighty thousand dairy producers participate in the dairy check-off program, which provides funding for promotion and research programs. The dairy check-off exists to help increase domestic and international demand for U.S.–produced dairy products. Since 1984 the check-off has been federally mandated. U.S. dairy farmers have to pay a fifteen-cent-per-hundredweight check-off on their milk production to be used for promotions (including the "Power of Cheese" campaign). Additionally, fluid milk processors pay a twenty-cent-per-hundredweight check-off for similar purposes (the "Got Milk?" campaign). Most major U.S. agricultural commodities have comparable mandatory promotional programs such as "Beef—It's What's for Dinner," the "Incredible, Edible Egg," or "Pork—The Other White Meat." Not all producers are happy with this federal mandate. On June 25, 2001, the Supreme Court ruled that the mandatory mushroom check-off violates the First Amendment free-speech rights of mushroom producers. In the fall of 2004, the court heard the beef check-off case, and is scheduled to issue a ruling sometime between March 15 and June 30, 2005.

2. USDA, National Agricultural Statistics Service, "Milk Production" (February 14, 2003), www.mannlib.cornell.edu/reports/nassr/dairy/ pmp-bb/2003/mkpr0203.txt.

3. USDA, Economic Research Service, "Organic Production" (Washington: USDA, 2002), www.ers.usda.gov/data/organic.

4. USDA, Agricultural Marketing Services, Pesticide Data Program, "Annual Summary Calendar Year, 1998" (Washington: USDA, 1998), 79.

5. John Robbins, *The Food Revolution: How Your Diet Can Help Save Your Life and Our World* (Berkeley: Conari Press, 2001), 107.

6. After the third time in twelve months, most state laws prohibit the offending farms from selling milk completely. *32.21 Adulterated dairy products,* subdivision 4, Penalties (c) (3), Office of Reviser of Statutes, State of Minnesota (2002).

7. John F. Beirbaum, Director, National Holstein Association, personal interview, November 25, 2002.

8. Ronnie Cummins, "BHG: Monsanto and the Dairy Industry's Dirty Little Secret," Organic Consumers Association, www.inmotionmagazine.com/ra02/geff13.html.

9. Julie Miller-Jones, College of St. Catherine, St. Paul, MN, telephone interview, May 2004.

10. USDA, Animal and Plant Health Inspection Service, National Center for Animal Health Surveillance, "Info Sheet: Bovine Somatotropin" (updated May 2003), www.aphis.usda.gov/vs/ceah/ncahs/dairy/Dairy02/Dairy02BST.pdf.

11. Ibid.

12. B. A. Crooker et al., "Dairy Research and Bovine Somatotropin," University of Minnesota (1994), www.extension.umn.edu/distribution/livestocksystems/DI6337.html.

13. D. M. Barbano et al., "Effect of Prolonged-Release Formulation of n-Methionyl Bovine Somatotropin on Milk Consumption," *Journal of Dairy Science* 75 (1992),

1775. Part of the difficulty of obtaining irrefutable evidence is that the amount of naturally occurring IGF-1 fluctuates with the cycle of the cow, her breed, and what she eats. Amounts range from undetectable to 30 ng/ml in an untreated cow. A study tested milk for IGH-1 and showed cows receiving rBST had levels of IGH-1 at 3.80, 5.39, and 4.98 ng/ml. Cows not receiving the hormone tested at 3.22, 2.62, and 3.78 ng/ml.

14. Dr. Samuel Epstein, "Unlabeled Milk from Cows Treated with Biosynthetic Growth Hormones: A Case of Regulatory Abdication," *International Journal of Health Sciences* 26, no. 1 (1996), 173–85.

15. "Monsanto Confirms Additional Cutback in Posilac" (January 23, 2004), www.dairyline.com/BST.htm.

16. Cooperatives Working Together (CWT) is a program within the National Milk Producers Federation that seeks to raise milk prices through buyouts of small, inefficient dairy herds. In 2003 CWT managed to buy out nearly two thousand dairy farmers and reduced the amount of milk production in 2004 by 608 million pounds. More information can be found at the CWT's website, www.cwt.coop/action/action_herd.html.

17. Ibid.

18. Malla Hovi et al., "Animal Health and Welfare in Organic Farming," College of Reading (January 28, 2001), www.organicvet.reading.ac.uk/Cattleweb/disease/mast/mast.htm. "Average individual cow SCC levels were significantly higher in Organic herds (135,000 cells/ml) than in Conventional herds (84,000 cells/ml; $P<0.001$), resulting in high sub-clinical mastitis levels in Organic herds (individual cow SCC> 200,000 cells/ml in 34% of all measurements)."

19. USDA, Agricultural Statistical Database, National Agricultural Statistic Service, "Milk Cow Herd Size by Inventory and Sales," Table 17 (accessed February 12,

2005), www.nass.usda.gov/census/census02/volume1/us/st99_1_017_019.pdf.

20. USDA, "Info Sheet: Bovine Somatotropin."

21. See www.junkscience.com/consumer/consumer_milk.htm.

22. G.F.W. Haenlein, "Goat Management: Alternatives in Dairy Goat Product Market," University of Delaware, http://ag.udel.edu/extention/information/goatmgt/gm-01.htm.

23. USDA, Agricultural Statistical Database, National Agricultural Statistic Service, "Milk Production, Disposition and Income, 2001" (accessed March 1, 2004), www.usda.mannlib.cornell.edu/reports/nassr/livestock/milk0402.txt.

24. General Nutrition Center, "Conjugated Linoleic Acid," www.bodyandfitness.com/Information/Weightloss/Research/cla1.htm#helps.

25. USDA, Agricultural Statistical Database, National Agricultural Statistics Service, "Chickens and Eggs Annual Summary, 2003" (accessed March 1, 2004), www.usda.mannlib.cornell.edu/reports/nassr/egg/pdp-bb/2003/egg0403.txt.

26. Bob Willis, owner, Cedar Grove Cheese Factory, Plain, WI, personal interview, November 2002.

27. Public Issues Education Project, Genetic Engineered Organisms, www.geopie.cornell.edu/crops/enzymes.html.

28. Tara Meissner, "State Can Expect to See More Dairy Cows," *Manitowoc Herald Times*, October 5, 2002, www.wisinfo.com/heraldtimes/news/archive/local_6403540.shtml.

29. Dairy Forum, "California Dairy Facts," www.dairyforum.org/cdf.html.

30. William Shurtleff and Akiko Aoyagi, *The Book of Tofu* (San Francisco: Autumn Press, 1975).

31. Valerie Freeman, "Oriental Odyssey," *Soil and Health* 61, no.4 (2002), 35.

32. Extoxnet, Extension Toxicology Network, Pesticide Information Profiles, http://extoxnet.orst.edu/pips/malathio.htm.

33. USDA, Agricultural Statistical Database, National Agricultural Statistics Service, "Chickens and Eggs Annual Summary, 2003" (accessed April 19, 2003), www.USDA.mannlib.cornell.edu/reports/nassr/poultry/pec-bbl/lyegan03.txt.

34. American Egg Board, Park Ridge, IL, www.aeb.org/eii/facts/industryfacts-06-2002.htm.

35. Rodger A. Ely, "An Investigation of the Extraction of Methamphetamine from Chicken Feed, and Other Myths," *Journal of the Forensic Science Society* 30 (1990), 363.

36. W. Gao et al., "Effect of Stocking Density on the Incidence of Usage of Enrichment Devices by White Leghorn Hens," *Journal of Applied Poultry Research* 3 (1994), 336.

37. Recommendations made by the NOSB are not official policy until they are approved and adopted by the USDA. See www.ams.usda.gov/nosb/index.htm.

38. USDA, National Organic Program, "Access to the Outdoors for Livestock" (October 29, 2002), www.ams.usda.gov/nop/NOP/PolicyStatements/LivestockAccess102902.pdf.

39. See Horizon Dairy's website, www.horizonorganic.com/about/farming.html.

40. John B. Carey and John T. Brake, "Induced Molting as a Management Tool," *Poultry Science and Technology Guide,* North Carolina State University at Raleigh (1987).

Aisle 5: Meat and Fish

1. Judith Putnam and Jane E. Allshouse, "Food Consumption, Prices, and Expenditures, 1970–97," Economic Research Service, *Statistical Bulletin*, no. 965 (Washington: USDA, 1999), table 1.

2. *The Jungle* set the standard by opening the slaughterhouse door; America peered in and recoiled in horror. Congress then leaped into action, passing the Pure Food and Drug Act in order to reassure the public that meat was safe to eat. Ever since, the public, Congress, and the livestock industry have been caught in this cycle: journalists write stories, people scream in protest, politicians offer soothing legislation. And each year, we consume more meat.

3. Corn as feed has been around a few hundred years, but soybeans are a recent addition. The USDA first listed soybeans as an agricultural commodity in 1925 when U.S. farmers raised 4.9 million bushels on 448,000 acres. By 2000, this number rose to 2.7 *billion* bushels on over 72 million acres. Soybeans are a legume and have more protein and fat than any other plant-based commodity. Livestock producers use this to their advantage, as both the fat and protein increase an animal's weight quickly.

4. Jim Riddle, "Why Organic Beef Is Safer than Conventional Beef," www.organicconsumers.org/organic/beef011204.cfm. The FDA banned the feeding of cattle brain and spinal tissue to cattle in 1997, but they still allow the following materials to be fed to nonorganic cattle: blood and blood products (from cattle and other species); gelatin (rendered from the hooves of cattle and other species); fats, oils, grease, and tallow (from cattle and other species); poultry and poultry

by-products; rendered pork protein; rendered horse protein; poultry manure (which may include spilled feed containing rendered animal products); and human food wastes (which may contain beef scraps).

5. Robert Cohen, "C Equals Crohn's Disease," www.not milk.com/c.html.
6. Some researchers connected to the organic community have developed a pesticide/copper deficiency/ sonic boom connection that challenges the established science.
7. The first three—estradiol (estrogen), progesterone, and testosterone—occur naturally. When hormone-treated cattle are tested, these natural hormones cannot be distinguished from those already in an animal's body, but tolerance levels are set according to the normal range of hormones found in an untreated animal's body. Zeranol, trenbolone acetate, and melengesterol are synthetic analogs of naturally occurring hormones and can be detected by testing.
8. See the Maverick Beef Ranch website, www.maverick ranch.com/factsmyths.htm.
9. USDA, Agricultural Statistical Database, National Agricultural Statistic Service, "Livestock Production, Disposition and Income, 2002" (accessed March 1, 2004), http://usda.mannlib.cornell.edu/reports/nassr/ livestock/pct-bb/cat10202.txt.
10. Sharon Durham, Agricultural Research Service, " 'Free-Range' Chicken—No Guarantee It's Free of *Salmonella*," (Washington, USDA, September 20, 2004), http://www.ars.usda.gov/IS/pr/2004/040920.htm.
11. Saskatchewan Pork Profile, www.collections.ic.gc.ca/ hog/info.html.
12. Rick Stock, "Feed Additives for Beef Cattle," University of Nebraska, www.ianrpubs.unl.edu/beef/g761.htm #esh.

13. Peter Lovenheim, *Portrait of a Burger as a Young Calf* (New York: Three Rivers Press, 2002), xii. Up to 70 percent of all processed beef products comes from downer milk cows or useless male calves.

14. A feedlot contains hundreds of small fenced-in plots (75 to 100 steers on an acre or less) that run along a feeding trough. The troughs run alongside a concrete driveway where ranchers deliver feed with a tractor. About once a month or so, workers push the manure from the plots into the center of the lot, forming a small mountain of dung.

15. See Eric Schlosser's *Fast Food Nation,* Upton Sinclair's *The Jungle,* Peter Lovenheim's *Portrait of a Burger as a Young Calf,* and John Robbins's *The Food Revolution.*

16. Christine Blank, "Organic Poultry and Egg Production Increases as Sales Heat Up," *Organic Business News* 16, no. 7 (July 2004), 6.

17. Ibid, 10.

18. See the Organic Valley website, www.organicvalley.coop/member/index.html.

19. John Fraser Hart, *The Changing Scale of American Agriculture,* (Charlottesville: University of Virginia Press, 2003), 211.

20. *CFR,* vol. 65, §205.239(C), 80646.

Aisle 6: Beverages

1. Bureau of International Labor Affairs, "By the Sweat and Toil of Children: Consumer Labels and Child Labor" (Washington: U.S. Department of Labor, 2000), www.dol.gov/ilab/media/reports/iclp/ sweat4/.

2. Swiss Import Promotion Program, "The Organic Market in Switzerland and the European Union—Organic Coffee, Cocoa and Tea," (January 2002), 96.

3. FDA, Total Diet Study (also called the Market Basket Study), www.cfsan.fda.gov/~comm/tds-toc.html. Foods found with lindane include a chocolate cake mix with .0002 ppm and a chocolate-coated candy bar with .00019 ppm.

4. Committee on Nutrition, "Policy Statement: The Use and Misuse of Fruit Juice in Pediatrics," *Pediatrics* 107, no. 5 (2001): 1210–1213.

Aisle 7: Processed Foods

1. John M. Connor and William A. Schiek, *Food Processing: An Industrial Powerhouse in Transition,* 2nd ed. (New York: John Wiley & Sons, 1997), 6.

2. Organic Foods Production Act, subsection 205.270.

3. Laurie Demeritt, "Consumer Trends in Organic," presentation at Organic Trade Association's All Things Organic trade show May 3, 2004.

4. *CFR,* vol. 65 §205.270 (b) (1), 80645.

5. Steve Meyerowitz, *The Organic Food Guide: How to Shop Smarter and Eat Healthier.* (Guilford, CT: Globe Pequot Press, 2004), 2, 6.

6. Kate Clancy and Fred Kirschenmann, "Keeping It Organic: Making Sense Out of the Processing of Organic Food," www.biotechinfo.net/keeping_organic.html.

Conclusion: Beyond the Checkout Counter

1. Erica Walz, "Final Results of the Fourth National Organic Farmers' Survey: Sustaining Farms in a Changing Organic Marketplace," Organic Farming Research Foundation (2004), 20.

Index

About the Authors

LUDDENE PERRY began her career in organics with a small plot in Colorado almost forty years ago. She is currently a teacher of horticultural food production and garden and landscape design, based in Minneapolis. She founded an organic-certifying company in 1992, and her innovations in the industry led to what are now standard certifying procedures. She is a member of the Independent Organic Inspectors Association and actively consults with the organic-processing industry.

DAN SCHULTZ is a freelance writer who began working as a structural pest control operator in 1988. He lives in Minneapolis.

From the Editors of *Prevention* Magazine Health Books

THE DOCTORS BOOK OF HOME REMEDIES

This complete, practical guide contains more than 2,300 accessible healing tips for the most common medical complaints, including bladder infections, depression, emphysema, headaches, PMS, toothaches, and much more.

___978-0553-58555-1 $7.99/$11.99 in Canada

THE DOCTORS BOOK OF HOME REMEDIES II

The sequel to the bestselling *The Doctors Book of Home Remedies*, with more than 1,200 all-new doctor-tested tips anyone can use to heal everyday health problems.

___978-0553-56984-1 $7.50/$9.99

THE DOCTORS BOOK OF HOME REMEDIES FOR CHILDREN

For the first time, here is complete, time-tested home remedy advice for child health care, from infancy through age 12.

___978-0553-56985-8 $6.99/$8.99

THE DOCTORS BOOK OF HOME REMEDIES FOR DOGS AND CATS

This book offers the best advice on the emotional and physical health of dogs and cats, gathered from more than 200 experts.

___978-0553-57781-5 $7.50/$10.99

From the Editors of *Prevention* Magazine Health Books

Guía Médica de Remedios Caseros

The Spanish-language debut of the indispensable volume of informative at-home remedies.

___56986-4 $7.50/$10.99

The New Healing Herbs

This comprehensive guide to medicinal plants contains all the information readers need to use them confidently, effectively, and safely—including an A-to-Z encyclopedia of 100 herbs and remedies for more than 100 common conditions.

___58514-2 $7.99/$11.99

Symptoms: Their Causes and Cures

You have a pain or an ache, a tingling or a rash. You know it's your body's way of telling you that something is wrong—but what? SYMPTOMS is an easy-to-use A-to-Z guide to 265 of the most common symptoms—and what they mean.

___56989-9 $7.50/$9.99

....

Please enclose check or money order only, no cash or CODs. Shipping & handling costs: $5.50 U.S. mail, $7.50 UPS. New York and Tennessee residents must remit applicable sales tax. Canadian residents must remit applicable GST and provincial taxes. Please allow 4 - 6 weeks for delivery. All orders are subject to availability. This offer subject to change without notice. Please call 1-800-726-0600 for further information.

Bantam Dell Publishing Group, Inc.	TOTAL AMT	$_____
Attn: Customer Service	SHIPPING & HANDLING	$_____
400 Hahn Road	SALES TAX (NY, TN)	$_____
Westminster, MD 21157		
	TOTAL ENCLOSED	$_____

Name _____

Address _____

City/State/Zip _____

Daytime Phone (_____) _____

*"A comprehensive up-to-date compendium of useful
advice on the health requirements for women."*
—*Gary Null, author of* GOOD FOOD, GOOD MOOD

SUPER NUTRITION
FOR WOMEN

A FOOD-WISE GUIDE FOR HEALTH, BEAUTY, ENERGY AND IMMUNITY

BY THE AUTHOR OF *BEYOND PRITIKIN*
ANN LOUISE GITTLEMAN, M.S.,
WITH J. LYNNE DODSON

It is becoming more and more evident that many of the so-called "healthy" diets, even the currently popular high-carbohydrate, low-fat diets, are designed with men in mind—and a woman cannot be healthy on a man's diet. Now here's a scientifically based dietary program that takes into account a woman's special body chemistry and unique nutritional needs. *Super Nutrition for Women* shows how to strengthen your immune system and prevent and combat a variety of illnesses, including yeast infections, premenstrual syndrome, osteoporosis, breast cancer, and coronary heart disease.

_____978-0553-38250-1 $15.00/$23.00 in Canada

Ask for this title wherever books are sold, or visit us online at
www.bantamdell.com for ordering information.

HN 15 2/07

The ultimate home reference from the diabetes experts

American Diabetes Association
Complete Guide to Diabetes
Revised 4th Edition

The American Diabetes Association has compiled this one-volume sourcebook to bring you the most up-to-date information you need to live an active, healthy life with diabetes. This comprehensive home reference gives you information on the best self-care techniques and latest medical breakthroughs.

"An indispensable new reference."
—*Consumer Reports on Health*

"A comprehensive, all-in-one guide to diabetes."
—*Pharmacy Times*

____978-0553-58907-8 $7.99/$10.99

Corinne T. Netzer

SHE KNOWS WHAT'S GOOD FOR YOU!